MAKE YOUR BODY A
FAT-BURNING MACHINE

Also by John Abdo

Body Engineering *(with Kenneth A. Dachman)*

Vital Living from the Inside Out

MAKE YOUR BODY A
FAT-BURNING MACHINE

30
DAYS TO A LEANER
AND HEALTHIER YOU

John Abdo

ST. MARTIN'S GRIFFIN ✹ NEW YORK

www.stmartins.com

Except where otherwise noted, all the charts and graphs were designed by John Abdo.

Photographs on page 8 (right) and pages 72–76 are by Jim Amentler.

Book design by Michael Mendelsohn

Library of Congress Cataloging-in-Publication Data
Abdo, John.
    Make your body a fat-burning machine: 30 days to a leaner and healthier you / John Abdo.
       p. cm.
    ISBN 0-312-28749-6
    1. Physical fitness. 2. Weight loss. 3. Health. 4. Nutrition. I. Title.
RA776 .A166 2002
613.7—dc21   2002024864

First Edition: September 2002

10 9 8 7 6 5 4 3 2 1

A Note to Readers

This book is for informational purposes only.
Readers are advised to consult a physician before making any major
change in exercise regimen or lifestyle.

To my daughter, Martina, who has inspired me with her courageous and enthusiastic efforts in winning her battle against obesity and transforming herself into a healthy, athletic, and beautiful young woman.

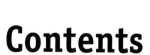

Contents

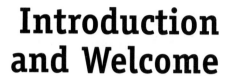

Introduction
and Welcome

It's lunchtime in a Rochester, Minnesota, diner less than a mile from the Mayo Clinic.

"What the heck is that?" Bud asks.

"The Tuesday Special," Lou replies. "A double-bacon cheddar burger and a side of curly Parmesan fries. It comes with this bright orange frozen thing."

"It should come with a defibrillator," Bud says.

Flash eighteen hundred miles west to a Las Vegas casino. Laverne and Shirley, their digestive systems still rumbling with toxic explosions ignited an hour earlier at the $3.99 Bountiful Bonanza Breakfast Buffet, are smoking and joking in the video poker bar.

"We gotta go," Laverne says as she drains her tequila sunrise. "Bingo starts in five minutes."

The television above the bar is tuned to ESPN. On the screen, a tan, toned surf sprite works out on a sand dune overlooking the Pacific Ocean.

Shirley fires up her sixth cigarette of the morning. "Let's roll," she says. "Little Miss Hard Body will have to party on without us."

Down at the end of a leafy cul-de-sac in Burlington, Vermont, Ward is cleaning his garage. A dusty cardboard box labeled EX STUFF is not where Ward believes it should be.

As he lifts the box, a sudden sharp pain four inches wide and very deep sears Ward's lower back. His arms go numb; he drops the box on his left foot; he collapses; he screams.

"June!" Ward shrieks. "Call . . . paramedics . . . quick!"

EX STUFF, June recalls as she sits in the emergency room's waiting area, is her abbreviation for exercise equipment. The box that brought Ward down contained dumbbells, boxing gloves, and assorted fitness paraphernalia that Ward hasn't used for at least three years.

Four pale stringy teens slouch on benches in the central atrium of a huge enclosed shopping mall northwest of Chicago.

"This sucks," says Lenny. He is wearing a *We Ain't Leavin' Till We're Heavin'* tank top. "There's absolutely nothing to do."

"The new Arnold flick's at the Cineplex," says Richie.

"Saw it," says Moose. "Man, that dude is awesome. His chest takes up the whole screen."

"Arcade," Eddie says. "You guys got any quarters?"

Across the road from the mall is a sixty-eight-acre nature preserve where miles of wide smooth bicycle trails wind gracefully through dark green forests and rolling grasslands.

On the rooftop of a Birmingham, Alabama, nursing home, Sylvia slumps in her wheelchair and gazes with obvious distaste at a brown skyline of smokestacks and grain elevators.

This is not the retirement Sylvia had in mind. She had planned to spend her golden years escorting her grandchildren around Disney World, cruising the South Pacific, and strolling the narrow stone streets of quaint European hamlets.

Instead, she lives in a chair.

Sylvia is barely seventy, but her body is much older. The bones in her legs are fragile, almost translucent, incapable of supporting her. And Sylvia's arms are too weak to propel her wheelchair from here to there. She must depend on others for even limited mobility.

"Ready, hon?" asks Troy, the attendant responsible for Sylvia and several other residents of the home's first floor. "It's getting to be time for your nap."

"Whatever," says Sylvia.

This concludes our program of selected short subjects (tentatively titled "Looking for Clues at the Scene of the Crime"). Sadly, these true-to-life Kodak moments pretty accurately portray the current state of health and fitness in the U.S.A. The average person of any age, of either gender, is in deplorable physical and psychological shape. One in four American adults is obese; more than half of us are overweight. Cardiovascular failures and other disorders directly related to poor eating habits and sedentary lifestyles are responsible for more than half the deaths in the United States each year. One of six American children is incapable of passing even the easiest physical fitness test. Medical expenses and lost productivity associated with what we eat and how we live drain billions from our economy each year.

I have a computer full of these alarming and depressing statistics, and I could go on, but I suspect that just about now you are muttering to yourself something like this: "Okay. Put away the two-by-four. I'm not an idiot. I get it. Our bodies are a mess. We're ruining our insides and shortening our lives. We're evolving into a nation of puffy puny techno-geeks. In the not-too-distant future we'll have to invent machines to feed us and operate our lungs and pump our blood and turn us over in bed at night. We are in major trouble."

Yes, we are. But look around. How can that be?

If we look for health and fitness books at Amazon.com, our search will yield over thirty-one thousand titles. Dozens of fitness publications share space with the *Star* and the *Enquirer* in our supermarkets' read-while-you-wait racks. We can view scores of fitness videos featuring former pro athletes, ex–drill sergeants, supermodels, actresses, and exercise gurus. We can listen to audiotapes (standard, evangelical, or subliminal). We can enrich, supplement, control, or turbocharge our diets with pills, powders, potions, and sublingual sprays. We can coat our tongues with a chocolate mist and convince our brains that we've just mainlined a kilo of fudge. We can join health clubs, spend our vacations at spas and boot camps, or hire personal trainers. We can buy machines—thigh melters, belly busters and tush tighteners, skiing simulators, stationary bikes, treadmills, stair steppers. We can climb concrete mountains or row down cartoon rivers. We can be hypnotized, aerobicized, nutrasized, pulverized, or jazzercized.

It's a little puzzling, isn't it? Despite the wealth of information, advice, and assistance available to most of its citizens, the U.S.A. remains the softest, roundest, fattest, and most depressed nation on earth. It's an annoying paradox. There are so many resources at our disposal. Why aren't we all fit?

Well, there are lots of reasons.

Many of the fitness products we buy quickly bore us or fail to deliver the amazing advances that their sales pitches promise. Many of the diet and exercise programs we try are fraudulent; their benefits vanish quickly or never appear at all. Some are too narrowly focused, concentrated within some ultimately meaningless band of the fitness spectrum. Others are too dogmatic, demanding a "my way or the highway" allegiance. Most are simply unrealistic, viable perhaps in a remote monastery or Foreign Legion outpost but completely impractical in twenty-first-century America.

A common failing of many diet and exercise regimens is a naïve reliance on deprivation and discomfort: "No pain, no gain." Most of us will not stay with a diet that denies us our favorite foods. Nor will we bust our butts at the gym for several hours a week, particularly if the results we're after seem too slow in coming. As soon as we discover the pleasure and freedom we experience when violating an overly restrictive fitness program's taboos, our rebellion begins. We drift back to our old habits. Yeah, we're still soft and weak, but, hey, we're free! Who wants to live to be ninety if it costs the equivalent of three decades in fitness prison?

Unfortunately, too many of us attribute our fitness failures to weaknesses within ourselves rather than to the shortcomings of boring or ineffective or impractical programs. And if we run the gauntlet of trial and failure often enough, the self-doubt and loss of self-esteem frequently associated with the misplaced blame we're piling up inside leads many of us to indifference or despair—and certainly to the conclusion that future efforts are useless.

Don't give up just yet. We're not doomed. I have an effective antidote for those intense blues. Drawing upon years of experience training world-class athletes, as well as hundreds of thousands of non-athletes, I've designed a comprehensive exercise and nutrition system you can use to burn fat safely and comfortably. And I promise that what I have to show you will work regardless of your age or size or sex. You're not too old or too fat or too weak or too far gone.

You will need to work on yourself, of course, but what I'm going to propose won't require superhuman effort. You won't need daily marathon sessions in the gym or expensive equipment or a health club membership. You won't be forced to replace real food with soy foam or sawdust pellets. You won't crush your spinal column or tear your arms from their sockets or blow up your lungs. And you won't be bored out of your mind or cheated out of your money.

You will control each aspect of your body's renewal.

And within thirty days your body will be leaner, stronger, and more efficient than it has ever been!

From Fat to Fit: The John Abdo Story

Hello, my name is Dr. Ken Dachman. I'm the author of several books and John's consultant on psychological variables in health and fitness. We've been working together over the past ten years to develop successful motivational strategies. I'm coming on stage for a brief moment because I believe that, in order to fully appreciate and accept the truly life-changing information John has to offer, you need to know who John is and, more important, how he became who he is.

I think John's story is an engaging, thoroughly American chronicle—real-life evidence that failure can be transformed into success, despair can lead to triumph, and error can evolve into enlightenment.

So here, culled from our numerous discussions conducted during this book's infancy, is John Abdo's story.

KD: Thousands and probably millions of people are currently using your programs and products to become or stay fit. That must be very gratifying.

JA: It is a wonderful feeling. I have men and women of all ages, occupations, shapes, and sizes who are seriously committed to improving their bodies and their lives. The testimonials I receive are nothing less than remarkable.

KD: You must be proud of what you've done for them.

JA: It is personally satisfying to be able to help, but let's not forget that their achievements are really theirs, not mine.

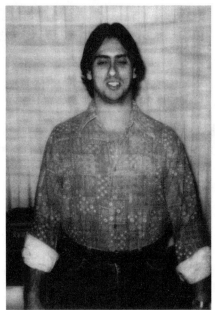 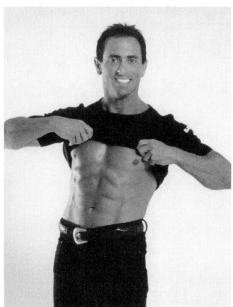

John Abdo: age 28, 215 pounds.   *John now.*

KD: I have a photo here. Who is this guy?

JA: That's me at twenty-eight, with fifty pounds of extra fat.

KD: No offense, but it looks like more.

JA: Well, I was only five feet eight. I had a 42-inch waist then and a rear end so big I had to wear size 46 pants. Huge thighs, too.

KD: What a transformation! Let's see. . . . You're forty-six, 165 pounds. You have a 32-inch waist and only 6 percent body fat. Is this accurate?

JA: Give or take an ounce here, a centimeter there.

KD: So we call your story what? Fat Kid to Fitness Superstar?

JA: Fat kid is certainly accurate. Fitness superstar sounds like infomercial hyperbole. I'd prefer to be known as a trainer, teacher, and motivator.

KD: Wouldn't "fitness expert" be a fair title? You have, after all, pretty much immersed yourself in the fitness field and related disciplines for the past thirty years.

JA: Yes, I have been doing this a long, long time. It's my life's work. And you know what? I love it. Especially right now. There's never been so much valuable data linking a fit lifestyle to longevity and good health. And there's never been so many effective methods for making all that information work for us. I've never been so confident about showing the average person how to become fit, trim, strong, and healthy.

KD: Where does that confidence come from?

JA: From what I know, of course, but more directly from what I've done. Sometimes I can talk an unsuspecting athlete into trying some new exercise technique or nutritional approach that I find interesting, but most of the time I test all my programs and products and recommendations on myself.

KD: So you're a living fitness lab?

JA: I guess so. I've been experimenting on myself since I was a kid—with no clue and a completely goofy plan initially, on purpose and with clear goals later on. I sometimes think I developed the saying "trial and error."

KD: When did all this start?

JA: When I was about twelve. I wanted to protect myself from street gangs, impress girls, and play football, so I started lifting weights. My dad, bless his heart, introduced me to weight training. But back then it wasn't really training. Nobody really knew about the links between weight work, diet, and metabolism, so Pop and I did what everybody did at the time. "Lift heavy and eat everything you can get your hands on" was our motto.

KD: A fine motto, but what were you trying to accomplish?

JA: I was trying to get really big and really strong. And I did. I also became slow, lazy, clumsy, and fat. Even though I exercised like a madman and swallowed what I thought were the right vitamins and supplements, I never came close to being fit or healthy. My exercise plan was to lift until my nose bled. My eating strategy was to wash down a dozen fast-food burgers with a bag of pretzels, a blueberry pie, and a vat of ice cream. Midway through most meals I'd have to unbuckle my belt and unzip my pants to make room for all the food I was shoveling down.

KD: I'm guessing that the results of this strategy were, um, interesting?

JA: You might say that. Bizarre is probably a better way to describe it. I made myself into a couch potato who was as strong as an ox. I could handle enormous loads in the weight room. I was really very strong. Unfortunately, there wasn't much call for curls or bench presses out in the real world. I didn't move very well, and the 20-inch neck I had developed often made it difficult to breathe. And, of course, I was fat—almost as wide as I was tall, with a huge spare tire and an enormous butt. And at some point in high school I cracked a vertebra.

KD: How long did it take you to overcome that terrible start?

JA: Years, actually. My first glimpse of what I might someday become came around 1973. I picked up some bodybuilding magazines that featured guys with a lean symmetrical look. I studied their training approaches and was surprised to find that careful attention to diet was an important element of their regimens. I tried several diets and even took weight loss drugs. The quick fix I was searching for never materialized. I spent the next twelve years buying almost every bodybuilding and diet supplement that came along. Man, did that get expensive. In the end I believe it was worth it. I learned what works and, maybe just as important, what doesn't. The people I train don't have to slog through the vast swamp of fitness programs and products out there; I've done it for them.

KD: At what point did you really begin to feel you had something valuable to offer as a trainer or teacher?

JA: When I became confident in what I was doing and when I began to see results—sustained improvements first in myself and then in my clients.

KD: And when did you achieve what you considered professional success?

JA: It took a while—years, in fact. When I began, I ran into a lot of skepticism, opposition, and outright rejection. There was a widespread misconception that average adults didn't need or benefit from exercise. A kind of medicine show, snake oil atmosphere tainted most vitamin and supplement ads. Mass marketing campaigns for bogus or dubious equipment were based on exaggerated claims or outright lies. All of this made it tough for legitimate fitness teachers to be taken seriously. The charlatans and hustlers cheated and disappointed so many people that it was tough to convince the public that any program or product was worthwhile.

KD: But you persevered. Did anything special keep you going, or were you just plain stubborn?

JA: A clear vision of where I wanted to be, a pretty good idea of how to get there, and the confidence that I could get there kept me from throwing in the towel. Topflight athletes rely on these same qualities, I've learned, and so do the ordinary men and women who succeed in reaching their fitness goals.

KD: You've trained many premier athletes. Among them are Bonnie Blair, the speed skater who won five Olympic Gold Medals, world power lifting champion Craig Tokarski, and several professional basketball and football players. Isn't it difficult to prepare all these different athletes for such diverse activities?

JA: Not really. The body is a marvelous machine—a work of art, really. Much more cleverly designed than anything we humans have come up with so far. Once you know how this machine's basic processes work, you can adapt and direct training to any physical purpose, any reasonable goal. Understanding that principle is what led me to realize that the same training techniques elite athletes use can be modified to work quite well for the rest of us.

KD: If you can, summarize your experience in terms of its relevance to the average man or woman who's dissatisfied with his or her physical condition and ready to do something about it.

JA: Okay. I don't think it's the usual "Hey, I did it, and so can you" cliché, although that element certainly exists. It took me years to change my body and my life. The road I took was long and tedious and littered with detours. The teaching and training I can provide now offers a much easier, much more direct path to health and fitness.

KD: What you're saying then is "I did it, and it took me decades. You can do it, too, if you'll commit to a thirty-day effort."

JA: Exactly. And the effort required isn't beyond anyone's capabilities. My experiences offer an additional message for adults who think they reached their physical prime in their late teens or early twenties. Comparing my body now, at forty-six, to the lump that occupied my couch when I was twenty-eight should convince anyone that age doesn't need to be a barrier to fitness.

KD: Let's say I wandered in off the street looking for some kind of fat loss or fitness program. And let's say, because I've tried various approaches with little or no success, that I'm skeptical. What would you say to me?

JA: I'd tell you to forget everything you know or think you know about diet and exercise and weight loss and physical health in general. I'd ask you to wipe the slate clean. And then I'd say that what I am about to teach you is the truth. What I am about to teach you works. What I am about to teach you will change your life for the better, forever. What I am about to teach you has been implemented successfully by millions of people around the world. Commit to a reasonable effort, set some realistic goals, and in thirty days you'll be well on your way to the best body you've ever had.

Why Are We So Fat?

Every few months the Surgeon General or the American Heart Association or the Centers for Disease Control or some similar organization updates us on the status of our nation's fat epidemic. Reports of these findings usually make the six o'clock news. Television news editors, firm believers that no news story can be told without pictures, always use these occasions to send camera crews out to shoot some footage of fat Americans. The standard technique seems to be: Set up a camera at waist level, and aim it at pedestrian traffic on any downtown street. In about three minutes the camera crew will have all the excess flesh it needs.

The sources of this unsightly, unhealthy, and, ultimately, lethal girth are easy to identify. Stone Age genetics play a part, certainly, but—in the opinion of most experts—modern lifestyle choices are our real nemesis.

Let's consider the biogenetic component of the problem first.

In late 2001, German researchers succeeded in isolating a gene that, they insist, "predisposes" about a third of us to accumulate and retain body fat. This gene, it turns out, has been around for as long as we have.

Early in our evolution as a distinct species, starvation was a serious everpresent possibility. Prehistoric man's cellular structure adapted to this threat to survival by hoarding nutritional reserves—in the form of fat. As civilization advanced, the need for these emergency energy sources diminished and eventually (in fully developed countries anyway) disappeared altogether.

Unfortunately, deep within the cellular control center of bodies in which the "caveman" gene remains active, it's still the dawn of time. An obsolete chemical protocol governs internal fuel management systems with an intracellular paranoia that hasn't been relevant for generations. In effect, some of us are stuck with Flintstones bodies in a Jetsons world.

As for the relationship between physical condition and lifestyle choices, we can again use a historical perspective. And we won't have to go back too far. Not very long ago we were strong, active people. The typical American workday consisted of twelve to fourteen hours of hard, steady exertion. Today, millions of us earn our livings at jobs that require no strenuous activity of any kind. And despite our whining about deadlines and commitments and overflowing in-boxes and unreasonable bosses and killer traffic and hectic schedules, most of us find ourselves with enough spare time to indulge a mysterious addiction to television or the Internet. On the average we spend twenty-one hours a week in front of the screen.

There were no doughnut outlets at Plymouth Rock, no hamburgers along the Chisholm Trail, no quesadillas for Lewis, no milkshakes for Clark. We used to grow our food or hunt it down. We ate fresh natural meats, grains, fruits, and vegetables. Our affection for greasy, rich, sugar-laden foods is a relatively recent phenomenon.

We have become an all-you-can-eat-and-all-you-can-watch society even though survey after survey shows we know better, and even though so many of us truly want leaner, stronger, healthier bodies.

Tooling Up

Our cursory review of the origins of American fat is intended to demonstrate that the thick, greasy substance that slows and clogs the bodies of millions is not some incurable alien plague or a punishment from God or the manifestation of some deep-seated emotional problem or a badge of personal weakness. Excess fat is simply a natural by-product of a natural biological process, a process we can control in much the same way that we can control the performance of any other machine.

You can upgrade your home computer by installing a faster, more powerful operating system. You can improve your car's efficiency by ridding fuel lines of carbon deposits and fine-tuning the engine. A new filter and wider, cleaner airways can make your old furnace seem new. The same renewal, renovation, and restoration principles can be applied to streamline and turbocharge the body's internal mechanisms.

Every element of the fitness system presented in the pages that follow is geared toward harnessing and maximizing your body's innate fat-burning capabilities. And you won't need a supermodel's diet or a decathlete's training regimen or six years on a psychiatrist's couch to build the trim, lean body you want. You will need some basic knowledge, a sincere desire to succeed, and a serious commitment to continuous positive action.

The human body is an incredible machine, blessed with amazing power sources; lightning-quick communication channels; its own pharmacy, chemical plant, and amusement park; a state-of-the-art data-processing center; and a huge capacity for work and play. Best of all, the body is resilient. It doesn't matter if indifference, neglect, or flat-out abuse has weakened your body's infrastructure or slowed its functions. The influence of that caveman gene those German guys found can be overcome and neutralized. You can significantly reverse years of damage and decay in just thirty days. If you begin with a respectful appreciation of your body's amazing operating systems, you'll have no trouble implementing my fat-burning program.

To begin your renewal effort you'll focus on your body's core processes. By improving the efficiency of your vital internal mechanisms, you'll spark a long-term chain reaction that will lead to significant improvements in performance and appearance. Most important, this "inside-out" approach will ensure that the gains you make won't diminish over time. Assuming you meet some simple maintenance responsibilities, the dramatic advances you'll achieve can be permanent.

The traditional formula for weight loss is simple and well known: Eat less, exercise more. While I can't dispute the accuracy of this bedrock principle of body math, I can—and do—question its relevance. I don't think that losing weight is a particularly worthwhile goal unless the weight lost is fat.

To lose fat we must increase the rate and efficiency of several intricate physical and chemical processes occurring constantly in trillions of cells within our bodies. I'll show you exactly how to harness and exploit these processes with a variety of exercise options and nutritional strategies.

When you finish this book, you will know all you need to know to reach your goal. Because there's no special food or equipment to buy, and no daunting investment of time or effort, you'll have only one major obstacle to overcome—a single but potentially formidable threat to your success: *you.*

The unique blend of attitudes, outlook, needs, and beliefs that make you whoever you are must be reshaped and redirected to accommodate your fitness goals. You want to change; you want to improve. But no change is possible until you choose to change, and no change will occur until you act on that decision. You must want to do what needs to be done, and then you must do it.

The techniques and strategies I recommend aren't difficult to understand or put into practice. Depending on your relationship with yourself, generating the motivation necessary to build the body you want may prove to be the toughest obstacle you'll face. To clear that hurdle you'll need to understand and accept an invaluable lesson learned early in their careers by thousands of elite athletes: Motivation must come from within.

For most of us, effective motivational techniques require a strong intellectual foundation. Not unlike Spock, Captain Kirk's ultrarational Vulcan sidekick on the starship Enterprise, we won't really make a commitment to action until we've completed a thorough cost-benefit analysis.

Fair enough. Take a moment to crunch the data relevant to the fat reduction program I'm proposing, and you'll quickly realize that what you'll gain clearly and decisively exceeds what you'll pay.

Costs

▶ a few minutes every other day for exercise

▶ some moderate changes in your eating habits

Benefits

▶ a longer, more productive life

▶ increased self-confidence

▶ lower blood pressure

▶ a leaner, sleeker frame

▶ more energy

▶ improved appearance

▶ greater resistance to stress

▶ significantly reduced vulnerability to dozens of deadly diseases (many of which are much easier to prevent than to cure)

▶ a greatly expanded choice of recreational activities

▶ deeper, more refreshing sleep

▶ more and better sex

Pretty much a slam dunk, wouldn't you say?

Unfortunately, because we're human, being able to recognize and accept the indisputable value of an activity usually isn't enough to sustain the desire and effort required to complete that activity. Earthlings not entirely in tune with their inner Vulcan require motivational power sources equipped with some emotional valves and gaskets.

Let's see if we can explore those emotional components without lapsing into psychobabble.

Desire. Motivation begins with a sincere desire to succeed. As NFL football coach Mike Ditka frequently reminded his players (at the top of his lungs, with flecks of saliva fouling his mustache): "You gotta wanna!"

Faith. You must be convinced that your fat reduction efforts will be effective. If your doubts aren't diminished by the assurance that the process I'm recommending is based on proven, widely accepted body science, remember that I'm not a retired actor or a marketing figurehead. I'm an experienced professional trainer. Fitness has been my livelihood and my passion for over thirty years. Trust me. I know what works and why.

Hope. Nobody can be motivated to pursue any course of action he or she believes to be futile. If you think your body is too far gone to benefit from any fat loss program, think again. Thousands of people in no better shape than you have become leaner and fitter following the principles I advocate. Make a reasonable effort, and so will you.

Responsibility. Recognize that you and you alone are responsible for the success of the improvement process. Welcome the challenge. See the effort you're about to undertake as a valuable opportunity. Trust yourself with the responsibility you're about to accept and realize that you have within you all the resources needed to reach your goals.

A Sense of Urgency. Unless you do something about it, the metabolic processes that determine how much of what you eat is stored as fat become slower and less efficient with each passing day. The longer you wait to awaken and recharge your body's fat-burning capabilities, the more difficult that renewal becomes. Change now or pay later.

Embracing Change. Even though life is a series of never-ending changes, many of us fear change. Despite a keen dissatisfaction with our current condition, a deep-seated resistance to change prevents some of us from making the improvements we know we must make. Psychologists tell us that change makes us apprehensive because change, even change for the better, always introduces elements of the unknown into our lives. Unknowns, these experts say, create anxiety and fear. Okay, I agree that changing comfortable living patterns can cause an emotional backlash in some people, but, come on, I'm not going to demand that you move to Tibet to spend the rest of your life eating goat hooves and pushing boulders up the slopes of the Himalayas. I'm asking you to find a few minutes every other day to exercise and to pay closer attention to what you're eating. If the prospect of change troubles you, you can lighten up right now: My fat reduction recommendations require no major lifestyle alterations.

Your orientation period is over. It's time to begin. We'll proceed slowly, one step at a time, one day at a time. Each phase of my fat-burning program will be explained. You'll find plenty of charts and illustrations to assist you in understanding the process. Do the work you know you need to do, and in about a month your body will become a fat incinerator—a lean, clean, healthy machine.

2

Personal At-Home Assessments

The simple tests and measurements that follow have been designed to help you chart your progress as you work through your fat reduction process. Two weeks from now, being able to see clear evidence of your advancement from the baseline you'll establish today will assist in deepening and sustaining your confidence and resolve. If indications of slow improvement, or (dare I say it?) backsliding appear, you'll know it's time to reexamine and refocus your efforts.

It's important to remember that these tests won't be graded. They are investigative exercises, more like an eye exam than a calculus final. As you may have noticed, your body is distinctly different from the body your neighbor or your boss or your favorite sports icon walks around in. And so are your fat reduction objectives, your lifestyle, and your vision of what your new body will look and feel like. The information you gain from your initial self-assessment is for your personal use only—the starting point for your fat-burning program. As you complete each test, record the results on the score sheet that follows; the data will be useful later.

Many experts base their definitions of fitness on strict mathematical formulas that measure heart rate, work capacity, or fat-to-muscle ratios. I

Personal Progress Chart

Date	Resting Heart Rate	Body Fat Percentage	Body Weight (bedtime)	Body Weight (waking)	Body Temperature	Activity Notes (exercise, sports, games, etc.) *	Results & Benefits (body, mind, life, etc.) **

* Record any notes regarding your activities.
** Record all of the benefits you're experiencing to your body, attitude, and life. Even small results are significant.

don't, and neither should you. While recognizing the value of objective standards (and invoking them when necessary), I believe that, for most people, being fit means having the strength and energy and endurance to do the things you want to do. When you're comfortable about the way you look and feel and move, you'll know it.

There's one last truth to consider before you begin your self-assessment. If your fat reduction efforts are even partially successful, today is the last time your body will look or feel as it does now. Recognize that fact and don't become discouraged if you are less than thrilled with your test scores. Radical improvement will occur rapidly.

Doctor, Doctor, Tell Me the News

The most accurate way to assess your current physical condition is to submit to a thorough physical examination administered by a qualified medical professional. Unfortunately, a comprehensive battery is also the least convenient and most expensive option.

Despite the cost, if you are over thirty and have been living a sedentary life for more than three months, I strongly recommend that you consult a doctor before launching your fat reduction efforts. If you're a heart patient, a stroke victim, a diabetic, or an asthmatic, or if you are afflicted with high blood pressure or clinical obesity, you absolutely must have your doctor's approval and supervision.

Those of you who find the idea of a complete physical impractical or undesirable should at least think about a basic blood analysis and stress test. These simple protocols will tell you and your doctor a lot about the state of your internal operating systems.

The Self-Administered Stress Test

Your everyday activities, from climbing stairs to carrying groceries to chasing your kids through the park, already provide you with a pretty accurate impression of your general fitness level. A simple home version of the stress test administered by many physiologists will help quantify that impression. While the results won't be as complete or as precise as the data available from the bank of diagnostic monitors the professionals use, what you find about your current physical condition will be extremely useful.

To make sense of your stress test results, you'll need to know how to measure your pulse rate. The best location for taking your pulse is the radial artery in your wrist. (While the carotid artery in your neck is easier to find, it often produces inaccurate readings.)

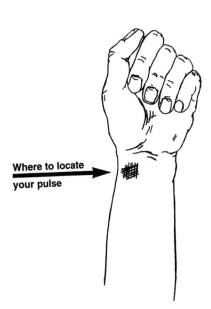

Where to locate your pulse

Locate your pulse using the sensitive tips of your middle and index fingers on your right hand. First find your wrist bone—it's at the base of your left thumb. Then move your fingertips toward your inner wrist until you feel your pulse in a pocket of flesh. Record your pulse beats for one minute to learn your "resting heart rate (RHR)." This "beats per minute" (bpm) number is a pretty reliable indicator of your body's cardiovascular efficiency. An efficient heart pumps more blood with each beat than an unfit heart, so the lower your bpm, the better:

Under 60 bpm	=	Excellent (10 points)
61–70 bpm	=	Good (5 points)
71–80 bpm	=	Average (3 points)
Over 80 bpm	=	Below Average (1 point)

The stress test you'll be performing measures how exercise affects your pulse rate. Because your pulse rate is an excellent barometer of heart and circulatory activity, your stress test results will demonstrate the impact of exertion on your body's cardiovascular infrastructure.

The STEP Test

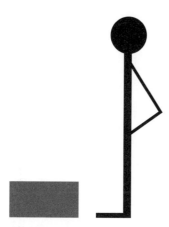

ONE: Place a sturdy box, or stool approximately 7" to 12" high in front of your body. Begin test by standing in front of the box.

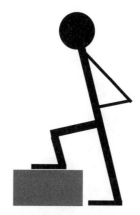

TWO: When you're ready to conduct your test, start the timer as soon as you lift your left leg—placing your left foot onto the box.

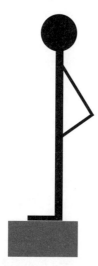

THREE: Follow your left leg with your right, so you're standing with both feet on top of the box.

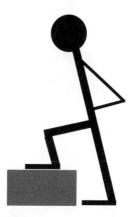

FOUR: After placing both feet onto the box, step down with the left foot first, then follow with the right. Repeat this left-leg up, right-leg up, left-leg down, right-leg down action as fast as you can for the duration of the test time. Upon completion, measure your pulse rate.

Resting Heart Rate

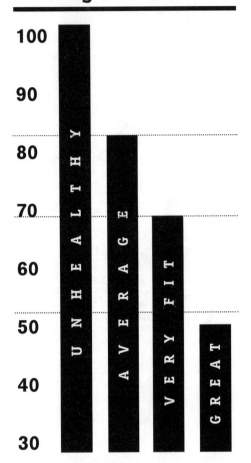

This graph illustrates resting heart rates (RHR), or beats per minute (BPM). Determine yours by taking your pulse for one minute. The best time to record RHR is first thing in the morning, prior to getting out of bed.

The home stress test is very simple, but it comes with a couple of important warnings:

IMPORTANT NOTE:
Do not take this test if your resting heart rate is over 100. Stop this test immediately if you experience dizziness, nausea, weakness, light-headedness, chest pain, or extreme shortness of breath. Sit down, recover, and see a doctor as soon as possible.

The test lasts one minute, so you'll need a watch, a timer, or some other way to know when a minute has elapsed.

1. Find a step, a sturdy box, or a bench 7 or 8 inches high.
2. Measure your pulse rate before starting.
3. Climb the step beginning with your left foot. Then bring up your right foot.
4. As soon as both feet are on the step, descend—left foot first, then the right.
5. Continue to climb (left foot), climb (right foot), descend (left foot), descend (right foot), etc., for 1 minute.
6. Count the number of times you bring up your left foot. Try to reach the count of 24 in the minute allowed for the test.
7. When your minute of exertion ends, sit down.
8. Wait one minute, then take your pulse. The number of beats per minute (bpm) will provide you with a glimpse of your cardiovascular fitness level and give you your first test score.

Less than 68 bpm	=	Excellent (10 points)
68–75 bpm	=	Good (5 points)
76–80 bpm	=	About Average (3 points)
Over 80 bpm	=	Below Average

An average or below average fitness level can be improved quickly—and significantly—by regular exercise. A good or excellent level suggests that you are either some kind of mutant or a person already involved in an active lifestyle.

Metabolic Tests

A useful gauge of the efficiency of several important internal mechanisms is your basal metabolic rate (BMR). Two simple tests will provide you with an adequate measurement of how well your metabolism is working.

Metabolic Self-Examination Chart

Day/Date	Bedtime BW	Morning BW	Weight Loss	Meals Notes	List of Activities	Retiring Measurement/s	Waking Measurement/s	Size Difference	Waking Temperature
EXAMPLES: Tuesday 8/20/02	183 lbs	178 lbs	5 lbs	5 meals total, Medium carbs	Weight training, 40 minutes on bike	Waist = 33"	Waist = 32"	Lost 1"	98.1°

Metabolic Self-Exam: Procedures: Weigh yourself before retiring, then again in the morning. Record both weights, and the difference between the two. Also measure any specific body area/s before retiring. Then again in the morning, record the difference. List activities, meals, and supplements from your day before retiring. Upon arising, before getting out of bed, place a thermometer under your tongue to record your body temperature. Readings between 97.8 and 98.6 are considered normal. Although temperature readings vary per individual, some authorities suggest that you can measure your BMR by consistently registering your morning or waking body temperatures. Readings below 97.8 are considered *hypoactive*, while readings higher than 98.6 are considered *hyperactive*. Those wishing to enhance and stabilize their metabolic rates–to speed the bodybuilding process and burn fat–should aim to set their temperature readings between 97.8 and 98.2, with occasional periods that exceed the higher limit, since intensive exercise will create higher than normal body temperatures.

In summary, the higher the body temperature, the higher the BMR, and this typically indicates a more active thyroid. However, unless you're suffering from an illness such as influenza, colds, etc, body temperature will rise during these bouts and is not healthy. Common factors that influence body temperature readings are the types and quantities of foods eaten, supplements, drugs, alcohol, coffee, mental state, stress, sleep, and exercise.

The Nocturnal Weight Loss Test

Weigh yourself before you go to sleep tonight and then again when you wake up tomorrow morning. If a weight loss of more than 2 pounds per 100 pounds of body weight has occurred overnight, your metabolic processes are working very well.

A weight loss of over 4 pounds (or 2.5 percent body weight)	=	Excellent (10 points)
3–4 pounds (or 2 percent of body weight)	=	Good (5 points)
1–2 pounds (or 1 percent of body weight)	=	Average (3 points)
Under 1 pound (or under 1 percent of body weight)	=	Below Average (1 point)

The Waking Temperature Test

If you wish, you can use a thermometer rather than a scale to measure your metabolic rate. Immediately upon waking (and while still in bed), place a thermometer under your tongue for ten minutes. A morning temperature high in the normal range of 97.8 through 98.6 is clear evidence of an active, efficient metabolism.

98.6 degrees	=	Excellent
98.2 degrees	=	Good
97.8 degrees	=	Average
Below 97.8	=	Below Average

Dysfunction Junction

The link between mental and physical health was established centuries ago in ancient Greece. Today, that mind-body connection is frequently the cause of serious physical ailments. The pace and pressures of modern life distract and disable us. This emotional stress creates degenerative imbalances in several life-sustaining internal systems. In fact, left unattended, emotional or psychological overload can lead to heart failure, stroke, and even death. Fortunately, as you'll learn shortly, the same emotional-physical conduits that allow what's happening in your mind to affect your body can be used to your advantage. Several elements of your fat reduction process will allow you to combat psychological stress with physical activities.

Unlike the cardiovascular stress we are able to quantify with the step test described earlier, emotional stress requires some subjective analysis. Twenty of the most common symptoms of stress are listed below. Note the symptoms you experience on a regular basis.

If five or more apply to you, you're living with too much stress.

If you are consistently exhibiting ten or more of these symptoms, please seek professional assistance immediately; your stress level is approaching a dangerous stage.

Symptoms of Emotional Stress

____ High cholesterol
____ Sexual dysfunction (impotence, lack of desire)
____ Rapid pulse
____ Loss of appetite
____ Nausea
____ Queasiness ("butterflies" in the stomach)
____ Frequent heartburn
____ Stiff neck
____ Sweaty palms
____ Frequent headaches
____ Insomnia
____ Chronic fatigue
____ High blood pressure
____ Binge eating
____ Chronic diarrhea or constipation
____ Teeth grinding
____ General anxiety or fear

___ Chronic irritability

___ Restlessness (can't sit still)

___ Indecisiveness

Less than 2 symptoms	=	Excellent (10 points)
2–3	=	Good (5 points)
4–5	=	Average (3 points)
6–10	=	Below Average (1 point)

Body Measurements

There are several reliable devices available to measure body composition and lean tissue levels. Your bathroom scale isn't one of them; however, you will use it on occasion.

As you work through the fat reduction process, there will be times when your weight seems stubbornly resistant to your efforts. Don't worry about it. Weight is an irrelevant indicator of progress. Muscle is heavier than fat, but muscle occupies less than one-third of the body mass that fat displaces.

To assemble your baseline body composition data, measure each of the areas indicated in the assessment chart. As you measure, be careful not to compress skin or flesh. Record these measurements, and at ten- or twelve-day intervals throughout your fat reduction process, use before-and-after comparisons to evaluate your progress.

Body Fat Ratio

Excess fat interferes with several of the body's most important functions and is the primary cause of most heart disease. Reaching and maintaining an acceptable body fat level is the primary goal of your fat reduction process. Our body fat ratio (not our weight) tells us how fat we really are. The 200-pound accountant with 26 percent body fat, for instance, is much fatter than a 240-pound linebacker of the same height who carries only 9 percent body fat.

Body Measurement Chart

DATE	Height	Weight	Neck	Shoulders	Chest	Bust	Waist	Hips/Buttocks	(R) Thigh	(L) Thigh	(R) Knee	(L) Knee	(R) Calf	(L) Calf	(R) Ankle	(L) Ankle	(R) Biceps	(L) Biceps	(R) Forearm	(L) Forearm	(R) Wrist	(L) Wrist

NOTE: Begin your fitness program by registering your complete body measurements. Once your initial measurements are recorded you can chart your progress by remeasuring each month. Enjoy the results month to month. Please make copies of this chart for repeated use.

There are a number of expensive "scientific" tests available to calculate body fat ratios. Unfortunately, most of them aren't nearly as accurate as their proponents claim they are. (The influences of intramuscular fat, gut gases, intestinal waste, tissue hydration levels, and so forth, are rarely accounted for correctly.)

The following tests will tell you all you need to know about your body fat level, and these tests, easily administered at home, cost nothing.

Women

1. Measure your hip girth at its widest point.
2. Determine your height (barefoot) in inches.
3. Using the chart, draw a straight line from your hip girth measurement (on the left) to your height (on the right).
4. Find the point at which this line crosses the (middle) Percent Fat scale. This point represents your body fat ratio.

Under 15 percent	=	Excellent (10 points)
15–22 percent	=	Good (5 points)
23–29 percent	=	Average (3 points)
30 percent +	=	Below Average (1 point)

Men

1. Determine your weight in pounds.
2. Measure your waist girth at its widest point.
3. Using the chart, draw a straight line from body weight (on the left) to waist girth (on the right).
4. Find the point where this line crosses the (middle) Percent Fat scale. This point represents your body fat ratio.

Under 10 percent	=	Excellent (10 points)
10–13 percent	=	Good (5 points)
14–19 percent	=	Average (3 points)
20 percent +	=	Below Average (1 point)

Calculating Body Fat Percentages

Women

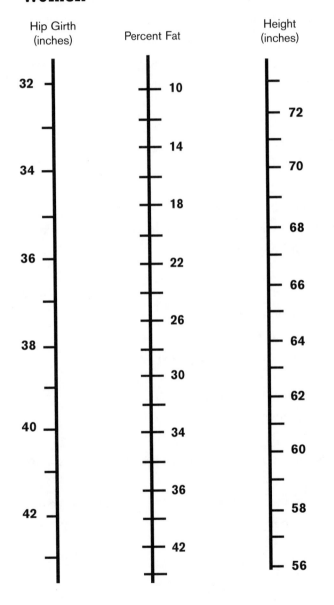

Hip Girth
(inches)

Percent Fat

Height
(inches)

PROCEDURE:
1. Record your height (without shoes): _____ inches.
2. Measure your hip girth at its widest point: _____ inches.
3. Go to figure and draw a straight line from your hip girth measurement (left column) to your height (right column).
4. Find the point where the line crosses the middle scale. This is your estimated percent of fat. Example: A woman with a hip girth of 38 inches who is 66 inches tall (5 feet 6 inches) has an estimated fat percentage of 27 percent.

Note: This chart estimates relative fat percentages in women based on body weight and abdominal or waistline circumference. ©1986 Jack H. Wilmore. Adapted and used by permission.

Calculating Body Fat Percentages

Men

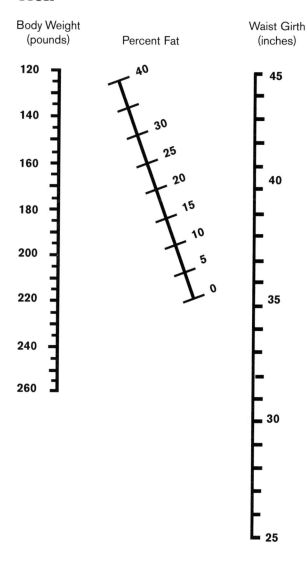

Body Weight
(pounds)

Percent Fat

Waist Girth
(inches)

PROCEDURE:
1. Record your current body weight: _____ pounds.
2. Measure your waistline at its widest point: _____ inches.
3. Go to figure and draw a straight line from your body weight (left column) to your waist girth (right column).
4. Find the point where the line crosses the middle scale. This is your estimated percent of fat. For example: a man who weighs 180 pounds with a 36 inch waistline girth has an estimated fat percentage of 18 percent.

Note: This chart estimates relative fat percentages in men based on body weight and abdominal or waistline circumference. ©1986 Jack H. Wilmore. Adapted and used by permission.

Fat Percentage of Total Body Weight

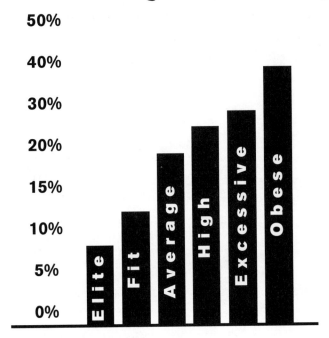

Endurance

Testing endurance is easy and in many cases not really necessary. If you find yourself short of breath after performing even moderately taxing physical activity, you already know you need to improve this aspect of fitness.

Endurance (or, as we big time trainers like to call it, "aerobic capacity") waxes or wanes as a function of your body's ability to process oxygen. Endurance deficiencies prevent the conversion of oxygen into usable fuel for the kinetic energy needed to sustain movement. Because expending energy through exercise is an important element in the incineration of body fat, you'll need to have—or be able to develop—at least a minimal level of endurance.

Perhaps the simplest endurance test involves a slow, easy jog. After a ten- to fifteen-minute warm-up (a short walk coupled with the stretching exercises detailed in Chapter 4 should be sufficient), jog for as long as you can without discomfort. Jog in place if you like or hit the road. When your body tells you it wants to stop, stop.

IMPORTANT NOTE:
Do not push yourself. Stop immediately if you experience dizziness, nausea, weakness, light-headedness, chest pain, or extreme shortness of breath. Sit down, recover, and see a doctor as soon as possible.

Compare the length of time you were able to jog with the general standards listed below for an approximate but adequate estimate of your current endurance level:

More than 30 minutes	=	Excellent (10 points)
20–30 minutes	=	Good (5 points)
10–20 minutes	=	Average (3 points)
Less than 10 minutes	=	Below Average (1 point)

Jump and Jiggle

Your final assessment exercise isn't at all scientific. It's a subjective visual aid—a kind of goofy but often helpful evaluation tool I call the Jump and Jiggle. Here's how it works:

Get as close to naked as you deem advisable, but wear a supportive bra or brief.

Stand before a full-length mirror.

Flex all your muscles.

Using short, rapid bounces, jump up and down. You don't even need to jump high enough to bring both feet off the floor. Just bounce.

As you bounce, telltale jiggling will pinpoint body areas where excess fat has accumulated. Note these problem areas for future observation.

Repeat every thirty days or so during your fat-burning process.

Critique what you see on these occasions objectively and honestly. Don't be surprised when these critiques become more and more positive.

Jump and Jiggle Test

	Date	Date	Date	Date	Date	Date	Date	Date	Date	Date	Date	Date
Neck-Chin												
Shoulders												
Chest												
Bust												
Bra-line (back)												
Waist (front)												
Waist (sides)												
Thighs (front)												
Groin												
Hamstrings												
Hips												
Buttocks												
Knees												
Calves												
Ankles												
Arms (front)												
Arms (back)												

There are various tests and procedures that can determine the percentage of fat on your body. In my opinion, many of these tests are inaccurate, expensive, and inconvenient. While standing stark naked in front of my bathroom mirror one day, I discovered a procedure that quickly located all of the fatty areas on my body. This fast and easy body fat test doesn't indicate exactly how much fat you have, but clearly points to where your fat is.

Here's how it works: Start by standing in front of a mirror with as little clothing on as possible. (For women, please wear a supportive bra and for you guys a supportive brief.) Stand upright and bend your arms at the elbows keeping them clenched to your sides. Tighten up your muscles as if a bucket of cold water was just dumped on you. While in this state of total body flexion, start to bounce slightly up and down without your feet leaving the floor. Look for whatever jiggles—it's that simple. If it's jiggling, then it probably doesn't belong there, and we'll make sure it burns away really soon!

C H A P T E R **3**

Adjusting the Fuel Mix: Easy, Nutritious, and Balanced Eating

Imagine this: Your doorbell rings. You open the front door to find a young man in a long white lab coat emblazoned with lightning bolts and geometric equations. He is carrying a clipboard and smiling benevolently. Although you've never actually seen him before, the man seems familiar. You speculate (accurately) that his father is a network news anchor, his mother a nuclear physicist. You guess (incorrectly) that his name is Zeus or Gabriel.

"I'm Bob," the man says. "This is your lucky day. I have something for you. Something very special. Come with me."

Intrigued, you follow Bob out to the street. Parked at the curb is the most spectacular automobile you've ever seen.

Bob hands you a set of keys. "It's yours," he says.

"What is it?" you ask. "The new Corvette model?"

"Could be," says Bob.

"No . . . wait. It looks more like a Jag," you say. "No, a Viper."

"If you want," says Bob.

You blink thrice and shake your head. "Hey, what's going on?" you ask. "Now I seem to be getting more of a Porsche vibe."

"Really," says Bob, not at all surprised.

"No, I was wrong," you say. "It's the Aston Martin from the Bond movies."

"Is it?" Bob asks.

"Maybe not," you reply, because now you're immersed in a rapid stream of Lexus, BMW, Rolls-Royce, and Lamborghini images.

Bob is a big fan of awestruck double, triple, and quadruple takes, but he has a schedule to keep. It's time to dispel your confusion.

"It will be whatever you decide it will be," Bob explains. "And it will run smoothly and silently for one hundred years. It's a classy complex machine with capabilities you won't even know about until you need them. Its state-of-the-art control center will regulate your speed, traction, and maneuverability. You'll never get lost; you'll always know the fastest, safest route to wherever you're going. You'll never find yourself stuck behind a smoke-spewing tractor-trailer or an octogenarian's Winnebago. You can drive this thing through hurricanes and avalanches, across lakes and up mountainsides."

"Cool," you say.

Bob nods. "The entertainment and information package provides concert-hall quality, digitally enhanced access to every piece of music ever recorded and a twenty-four-hour link to every broadcast outlet in the world. Fourteen hundred and six temperature sensors keep you as warm as toast in winter, as cool as a cucumber in summer. The onboard filtration plant scrubs, freshens, and sweetens every molecule of air you breathe. . . ."

As Bob continues in this vein, you circle the remarkable fantasy vehicle, trying your best to take in every aspect of its flawless chassis.

". . . and, of course, it will balance your checkbook, manage your stock portfolio, do your taxes, and pick up your dry cleaning," Bob says.

"Where's the gas cap?" you ask.

"There's no gas tank," Bob says. "The vehicle doesn't use gasoline—which, conveniently, brings us to your only responsibility."

"And that would be?"

"The car pretty much maintains itself," Bob says. "It keeps itself constantly tuned and lubricated, and it replaces virtually all its internal components every few months or so. All it needs from you is fuel."

Bob claps his hands sharply. The center of the vehicle's grille opens to reveal a funnel-shaped passageway.

"This is the fuel intake chamber," Bob says. "You'll need to fill 'er up every day or so."

"With what?" you ask.

"Well, that's up to you," Bob says. "The vehicle will run on almost anything flammable you choose to throw in there: charcoal briquettes, peat moss, cow chips, driftwood, whatever. But—"

"But what?" you ask warily. You knew there would be a catch.

"If you want to ensure that this amazing vehicle will continue to run at its optimum level for the rest of your life, you'll need to mix your own premium fuel," Bob says.

"Is that a big deal?" you ask. "It sounds like a big deal."

"Not really," says Bob. He hands you a laminated index card. "Just use this formula."

The instructions Bob provides are simple and easy to understand. Only one thing troubles you.

"You have some math happening here, Bob."

Bob sighs. "I get that reaction a lot. Let me tell you what I tell everyone else. Some people like the obsessively organized ultraprecise approach, but it's not really necessary. Forget about the ingredient ratios if they annoy you. You can eyeball the whole thing. Use a third of this, that, and the other. A sprinkle of additives if you like. That's it."

Okay, it's time to end our heavy-handed fable and make our point. One question ought to do it.

Would you be more likely to:

(a) follow Bob's fuel mix recommendations, or
(b) decide to power your incredible fantasy vehicle with a haphazard collection of old galoshes, Styrofoam cups, and whatever other trash you find along the road?

I know. It's a ridiculously easy choice. (Subtlety, if you haven't noticed, is not one of my strengths.) As you begin modifying your body's internal systems, you'll encounter a whole range of fuel choices just as obvious. And if our bodies were stand-alone machines like snowblowers or hydroplanes, or Bob's fantasy vehicle, most of us would have no trouble making and carrying out the correct decision.

Eating wisely is one of the most valuable things you can do for your body. That's a simple incontrovertible truth. You know it, but you also know that knowing it isn't enough. Our bodies and our psyches are closely and irrevocably intertwined. We can't ignore the role our mental state plays in nutrition. The rational core of our nature tells us that food is simply fuel, the only source of energy we need to sustain life. Cultural and emotional influences tell us something completely different, and, unfortunately, these powerful variables often play a dominant role in determining how and why we eat.

Too many of us treat food as an indulgence, a reward, a crutch, or a friend. In our affluent society, food is inextricably linked with sensory pleasure and social ritual. We celebrate important occasions by going out to dinner or attending parties set amid lush landscapes of rich, heavy food. Food is a gesture of welcome, warmth, hospitality. No social function seems complete or successful without it.

For too many of us, food becomes an addiction, an escape from boredom, loneliness, anxiety, or depression. Too many others find too much comfort in food or too much sensory pleasure.

Your body needs food to keep itself alive, to sustain thousands of mental and physical functions, and to construct or repair vital tissues. If you *need* food for any other reason, an important element of your fat reduction process has to be concentrated effort to free yourself of those entanglements.

Eating Strategies

The eating strategies I'll recommend to accelerate the fat-burning process require some common sense, some control, and some focus, and an understanding of how what you eat affects your body's operational performance. I won't ask you to agonize over food choices. Nor will you be required to weigh your food or count calories and/or fat grams. To prevent boredom and ensure that your body gets all the nutrients it needs, I will ask you to develop a realistic meal plan incorporating several food groups in proper proportion.

Let's begin to put together an effective and realistic eating strategy by examining and evaluating our core ingredients.

Proteins

The word *protein* is derived from the Greek *proteios,* which translates as "of the first importance." Aptly named, protein is, in fact, the basic building block of all living tissue. Your eyes are protein, so is your heart and liver, and so are your kidneys. Most of your body's cells are protein based, and protein is the primary component of muscle.

The value of protein can't be overstated. Your body's cells don't really live very long. With the exception of certain nerve cells, your cellular infrastructure is constantly in a state of regeneration. Protein provides the raw materials needed to sustain all the repair and renovation projects that keep the body alive by constantly building new tissue.

Deprive your body of protein (as many low-calorie diets do), and you'll quickly become grouchy, listless, tired, and weak. Your blood pressure will drop precipitously, and your resistance to infection will decline. Prolonged protein deprivation often leads to the breakdown of lean muscle tissue and may even cause kidney and liver failure.

Amino acids are the basic components of all proteins. Your body can't really use fully assembled protein molecules until internal processes break these molecules down into amino acids, which can be absorbed into the bloodstream. The body then selects the specific amino acids it needs for growth, construction, and repair functions. Of all the amino acids there are only nine that the body cannot make itself. These are called *essential amino acids.*

When it comes to supplying the body with essential amino acids, all proteins are not created equal. "Complete" proteins, such as meat, fish, poultry, eggs, and dairy products, offer adequate stores of the essential amino acids; "incomplete" proteins, such as those found in green and yellow vegetables, don't. According to recent studies, however, soy might be the world's first complete protein from nonanimal sources.

Fortunately for vegetarians and others interested in obtaining the benefits of protein, without having to deal with the blanket of animal fat in which a lot of proteins are wrapped, the body's internal chemistry lab can combine two or more incomplete proteins to develop a complete protein molecule.

The nature of protein and its central role in the metabolic process will be an indispensable ally in your fat reduction efforts.

Carbohydrates

Carbohydrates are chemical compounds made up of carbon, hydrogen, and oxygen. The smallest, simplest carbs, including glucose, come from foods such as fruit, table sugar, and pastries. Because glucose circulates through the bloodstream to deliver energy to the body's cells, this basic carbohydrate unit is also known as blood sugar.

Complex (or starchy) carbohydrates come from foods such as potatoes, bread, and pasta, which contain glucose molecules linked together in long chains of hundreds of molecules. Because of their size and structure, these giant carbs break down slowly—providing energy for extended periods of time.

Fibrous carbohydrates from carrots, celery, and other vegetables are rich sources of vitamins, minerals, enzymes, and of course, fiber.

> **An important point: Carbohydrates are the body's preferred energy source during exercise. Your body will burn fat only after it has depleted its available carb resources.**

If carbohydrates are such vital nutrients, you may wonder, what's the deal with the frequently (and loudly) repeated warnings that carbs are fattening, unhealthy, and dangerous?

The deal is that health and weight problems typically attributed to carbohydrate consumption are really an indictment of ill-advised, negligent, or just plain dumb eating patterns, not a condemnation of the nature of carbohydrates. If we overdose on any class of carbs and at the same time ignore our body's need for protein and other nutrients, our lean tissues will soon waste away, and we will become fat very quickly.

Judicious use of carbohydrates is obviously an important element in your fat reduction process. Any eating plan that doesn't acknowledge and accept the value and variety that carbohydrates offer is unrealistic and doomed to failure. So is any strategy that fails to deal with the dangers of reckless carbo consumption.

Fats

It turns out that dietary fat is not as evil as we thought, though some dietary fats are nastier than others and one class of fat is downright benevolent. Overindulgence in saturated fats (such as those found in prime rib and butter) or fats thick with trans fatty acids (such as the "partially hydrogenated" oils found in cookies and snack chips), for example, does indeed carry significant health risks. Pure monounsaturated (so called "good") fat—found in nuts, virgin olive oil, and avocados—on the other hand, may be one of the healthiest things you can eat.

Recent studies at Pennsylvania State University indicate that diets high in monounsaturated fat reduced heart disease risk by 25 percent. Additional research links monounsaturated fat consumption to higher testosterone levels in men, increased endurance in runners, and lower LDL (bad cholesterol) readings in general.

You'll probably want to reap the benefits that "good" fat has to offer, not simply because of your deep commitment to better health but because a lot of the stuff made with body-friendly fats really tastes good.

The Magic Formula

Now that we've established a general understanding of the basic ingredients we have available, we can begin to put together an effective fuel mix that you'll use for the next thirty days. Our objective? To kick-start your fat-burning process.

Let's start with a helpful graphic. The illustration on page 45 is supposed to represent a dinner plate—a regulation dinner plate, not a pizza pan or a trash can cover. You will notice that the plate is divided into thirds, depicting the balanced meals so helpful to the fat-burning process. When filling your real-life plate, use a mix of one-third protein, one-third fibrous carbs, and one-third starchy carbs. (You can have all the simple carbs you want once a day. More on that shortly.) Refer to the Nutrition Categories chart that begins on page 46 to select suitable foods for each third of your plate. Eat reasonable portions of each food you select. If you're still hungry when your plate is clean, go back for more, but please don't stuff yourself. However, you must balance those second helpings with foods from each group.

Use the approach that the plate represents as a baseline eating strategy to efficiently meet all your body's energy needs. You needn't concern yourself with calorie counts or fat grams or food weights. Nor does it matter what foods you choose from each category. Eat what you like but maintain the balance.

I strongly recommend a departure from the core eating plan once a day. At breakfast and lunch, stick to the three groups and nothing else. But at *dinner*, add starchy carbs such as potatoes, some bread (with butter, if you like), a cocktail, and dessert. Remember: Anything goes as long as you eat equal portions of the basic three food groups: protein, complex (starchy) carbs, and fibrous carbs. (See the Nutrition Categories again.)

This "window of opportunity" during which you can eat absolutely anything you want is provided to allow you the flexibility and freedom you'll need to sustain the long-term success you're striving for. You "pay" for this window of opportunity by eliminating or severely restricting your consumption of simple carbs during the day.

If the phrase "eat absolutely anything you want" plunged you into some twisted éclair and cheese block fantasy, snap out of it and straighten up. Your Window of Opportunity (W/O) Meal is subject to some specific but, I promise, completely reasonable guidelines. These restrictions exist not to annoy you but to help you regulate some potentially volatile aspects of your body's fuel management system.

Designing Nutritionally Balanced "Fat-Burning" Meals

Sample Meal

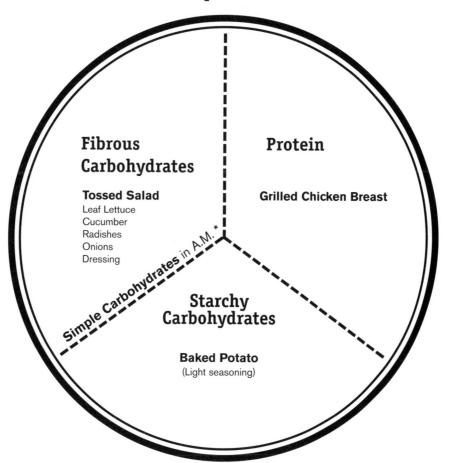

Designing balanced "nutrition-packed" meals is easy and fun when you follow my simple principle.

Explanation: Let's view the diagram above as a standard-size dinner plate. Start by dividing your plate into three equal parts. Once you've divided your plate, place a **Protein** food in the first third of the plate, then a **Starchy Carbohydrate** in the second third, and a **Fibrous Carbohydrate** in the final third. It's that simple!

* Simple Carbohydrates are another food category that may be included in your W/O Meal.

Refer to the Nutrition Categories chart provided in this book or simply make your own selections.

Nutrition Categories

Proteins

Foods containing essential and nonessential amino acids such as fish, turkey, chicken, lean red meat, soy, and eggs.

Carbohydrates

Simple Carbs: These are commonly referred to as monosaccharides and disaccharides; "mono" means one and "di" means two. Typically, simple sugars should be eaten earlier in the day for those trying to lose body fat, to allow the body the entire day to burn off those extra sugar calories before they convert into fat cells. Examples of simple carbs include grapefruit, plums, strawberries, apples, blueberries, and oranges.

Starchy Carbs: These food items, also known as complex carbs, contain sugar molecules (glucose) that are linked together in long chains known as polysaccharides; "poly" means many. These foods supply the body with a sustained energy source and are found in beans, rice, oatmeal, potatoes, pasta, rye bread, whole wheat bread, and muffins.

Fibrous Carbs: These food items contain inert carbohydrate molecules known as cellulose (plant sugars). However, too many raw fibrous carbohydrates can be detrimental to a sensitive digestive system. Fibrous carbohydrate foods should be steamed until soft, but not overcooked. Examples of fibrous carbs are broccoli, cauliflower, cabbage, leaf lettuce, onions, and radishes.

Fat

Saturated Fat   Bad fat!

These fats are typically hard at room temperature much like animal fats, creams, and butter.

Polyunsaturated Fat   Bad fat!

These fats are typically liquid at room temperature. Processed oils and margarines fall into this category.

Hydrogenated Fat   Bad fat!

These fats are produced through a process that takes previously good fats and destroys them in an attempt to extend their shelf life. Typically, these are hidden fats found in baked products like breads, muffins, and chips.

Monounsaturated Fat   Good fat!

Many oils such as olive oil and sunflower oil, as well as avocados, should replace other bad fats whenever possible.

Nutritional Guideline
Sample listing*

Proteins
Cheese (low or no fat)
Chicken
Cottage cheese (low fat, low sodium)
Eggs
Fish
Meat (lean red)
Shellfish
Turkey

Carbohydrates (Starchy or Complex)
Beans
Cereals
Corn
Crackers
Muffins
Oatmeal
Pancakes/Waffles
Pasta
Potatoes
Rice
Rye bread
Whole wheat bread (100 percent)

Carbohydrates (Fibrous)
(Mostly vegetables)
Alfalfa sprouts
Beets
Broccoli
Cabbage
Carrots
Cauliflower
Cucumber
Leaf lettuce
Mushrooms
Onions
Radishes
Tomatoes

Carbohydrates (Simple)
(All fruit)
Alcohol
Apples
Banana
Blueberries
Cantaloupe
Cherries
Dates
Figs
Grapefruit
Grapes
Ice cream
Melon
Oranges
Papaya
Pears
Peaches
Pineapple
Plums
Raisins
Sherbet
Strawberries
Yogurt

Beverages
Coffee/Tea
Fruit juice
Milk
Soft drinks
Vegetable juice
Water

*For an extended list of foods and serving sizes, consult *The NutriBase Complete Book of Food Counts* by Dr. Art Ulene.

First, you must begin your W/O Meal with a salad of greens and veggies. Some lettuce, asparagus, bean sprouts, radishes, green peppers—whatever you like from the fibrous carb category of the food chart.

Second, your W/O Meal must remain balanced. You can't use your window of opportunity to eat like an escaped con ransacking a bakery.

Start with reasonable portions of each food type. If you're still hungry after you've finished all the food on your plate, feel free to go back for more. Your second helping, be it large or small, must be equal portions of each food. Don't overload on the cake without sufficient proteins and veggies for counterbalance.

Finally, your Window of Opportunity Meal can remain open for only one hour a day. (You choose the hour.)

The principles behind this kick-start eating plan are solid and, judging from the impressive results I've seen so far, quite effective. The salads and other fibrous carbs you'll be eating regularly lower blood sugar and improve digestion. The proteins build muscle, organs, and other vital tissues. The simple carbs provide energy, satisfaction, and (usually within days) freedom from the fat and sugar cravings responsible for much of America's excess girth.

Speaking of fat, you may have noticed that our meal plan has no dietary fat compartment. That's because you'll get all the fat you need from your proteins and dressings. Recently, the American Heart Association commented that almost all of us are well aware of the link between excess dietary fat and a long scary list of diseases, and that the majority of us are sick of hearing about it. Okay, you know the overconsumption of dietary fat is stupid and dangerous. I know you know that. Do I really have to tell you to be sensible about the amount of fat you eat? I didn't think so. (Sensible, by the way, means less than 30 percent of your daily *food* intake.)

A typical day's menu might include a mushroom and green pepper omelet for breakfast; a turkey sandwich with mixed greens for lunch; and a Window of Opportunity Meal of salad, chicken, mashed potatoes with gravy, asparagus spears, and low-fat ice cream. Those of us who enjoy a glass of wine or a beer with dinner would certainly be able to do so—as long as we limit the entire meal to no longer than one hour.

The eating strategy I'm recommending to you establishes a nutritional balance and a predictable intake frequency that your body will quickly learn to appreciate. You can have the satisfaction of eating the foods you love, control your simple carb cravings, and heighten your body's fat incineration capabilities. An excellent deal.

Here's how the eating plan delivers its substantial benefits:

When you snack on simple carb foods and beverages all day, your body's internal control centers assume that each new meal or snack coming along will contain more of the same. In anticipation of another sugar delivery, your body releases a surge of insulin every time you eat. Because food was so scarce at the beginning of man's evolutionary history, our bodies were designed to conserve as much energy as possible during the nutritional process. The hormone insulin plays a key role in this conservation effort.

Among the many wonders of the human body is the speed and efficiency with which cellular structures react to stimuli. In the insulin production process, unfortunately, your body's quick response capabilities work against you. The more often you eat foods laced with simple carbs, the more insulin your body secretes every time you eat. This cycle of excessive simple carb ingestion/insulin spike is known as "maladaptive behavior," a condition associated with higher levels of sugar being stored as fat.

The window of opportunity eating strategy, in deference to this fact of biochemical life, restricts simple carb consumption to an hour a day and, even then, only in combination with complex carbs and proteins. The end result is a lower insulin response each time you eat.

The one-hour time limit imposed on your W/O Meal is also geared to modify and moderate your body's insulin management protocols.

From the moment the grizzly bear wakes in the spring until hibernation time the following winter, it spends every waking hour eating everything it can get its claws on. Our prehistoric ancestors, out of necessity, subscribed to the same nutritional philosophy. On the infrequent occasions when they stumbled upon plentiful food supplies, our cave-dwelling predecessors ate as much as they could for as long as it took. If two or four or seven hours were required to empty out a beet patch or a pomegranate orchard, so be it.

Way back then our body's fuel management systems learned that an initial surge of insulin wasn't always sufficient. The longer it takes to eat, our ancestors taught our cellular structures, the more we'll be eating. A second phase—a steadier, longer-lasting release of insulin—was quickly developed to cope with these consumption marathons.

Many twenty-first-century folk experience this secondary insulin release phase most noticeably on Thanksgiving Day. We begin eating at the first glimpse of the lead float in the Macy's parade, and we keep eating until the final whistle of the evening's football game. Strangely, the more we eat, the less satisfied we feel. The second wave of insulin that our daylong feast has stimulated is responsible for this nutritional contradiction.

The slow, steady second phase of insulin release typically reaches its peak about seventy minutes after we start eating. This explains why your window of opportunity is open for only an hour.

A fuel management system programmed to consume and hoard energy supplies at every opportunity made perfect sense during mankind's earliest days on earth. Today, with virtually limitless fuel sources so readily available to most of us, these obsolete processes can be burdensome and often dangerous unless we follow a nutrition plan designed to help us cope with the internal reactions that our eating habits provoke.

Feel free to nudge and tweak my recommended eating strategies to suit your individual preferences, but please stay within the boundaries I've established. Soon (usually within days) you'll notice a significant decline in sugar cravings and a marked increase in energy levels.

Let me stress that the program I've outlined here is not necessarily the nutrition plan I expect you to live with for the rest of your life. Once you've converted your body to the fat-burning machine I know it can become, you'll be free to customize your own strategies. (And the maintenance recommendations in Chapter 7 will help you do just that.)

The Snack Question:
Carbohydrate Addiction or Inattentive Eating?

If you spend a couple of days in a business office or shopping mall observing the natives' eating habits, you can easily conclude that we Americans are a nation of snack fiends. Doughnuts, bagels, or cinnamon rolls between breakfast and lunch. Cookies or ice cream or pizza bread between lunch and dinner. Chips, pretzels, or cheese spread before bed. Can so many of us really be that hungry all the time?

Of course not.

Much of this unnecessary eating is evidence of distraction or indifference. If one of our coworkers has a birthday or an anniversary and a cake appears, we have a piece. We kill time before a meeting with a croissant. Coffee breaks include a vending machine pastry because the coffee and pastry machine are there side by side. On days when we're busy, we'll eat whatever is easy, quick, and not too far away from our desks. If someone offers us food, we eat it whether we're hungry or not. In short, we're not paying attention. (The excess fat we accumulate with this lack of focus truly does sneak up on us.) Once recognized, snacking behavior attributable to this kind of general cluelessness is relatively easy to eliminate. The level of attention required to solve the problem is, after all, nowhere near as intense as the focused concentration needed to survive a midnight sleet storm on Route 66. It's more like the casual vigilance that keeps us from shredding the petunias or decapitating baby bunnies when we mow the lawn.

Typically, inattentive snackers wake up, remember that they are seriously involved in a heavy-duty fat-burning effort, and realize that swallowing every random edible within one's field of vision is probably going to make the whole fat reduction process a lot harder than it needs to be. (And that's exactly what should happen, don't you agree?)

Carbohydrate addiction is the complete opposite of inattentive eating. Comparing a carbohydrate addict to a distracted eater is like comparing a social drinker to a full-tilt alcoholic. Driven by a biochemical imbalance, carbohydrate addiction sparks a compelling hunger for sugar-rich foods. The ever-escalating, constantly recurring craving for high-carb junk overwhelms the addict, creating insulin overload and volatile changes in blood sugar levels, hence the term maladaptive behavior. For the carbohydrate addict the intensely felt need to snack furiously all day has a behavioral origin, in which the body's cravings override or control the mind.

There's good news if you suspect that you are a carbohydrate addict: The nutritional principles I've outlined will ease and perhaps eliminate your dependency.

Fuel Additives

Even when our meals are carefully planned and correctly balanced, the food we eat is often incapable of providing 100 percent of the nutrition the body needs to replace the energy resources expended in meeting the physical, social, occupational, and emotional demands of everyday living. In recognition of this cold hard fact, and to accelerate your fat reduction process, you may want to include nutritional supplements in your eating plan.

Before we discuss supplements, let's remember that fresh, healthy food is the foundation of effective nutrition. Swallowing fistfuls of pills isn't going to offset goofy eating strategies. Actual food must be and should be your primary nutritional and energy source, but it may be unrealistic to expect that you can meet all your body's needs without a supplement or two.

The problem is, many modern food sources have been stripped of natural nutrients. We're consuming packaged and processed foods that are far inferior to the staples harvested from the mineral-rich fields and forests of yesteryear. The actual nutritional benefit now found in many of our foods (especially grains, fruits, and vegetables) is significantly lower than it was when our grandparents were growing up.

To assemble all the nutrients your body needs from today's foods you'd have to eat all day, every day. That's obviously a dangerous impractical approach, so after installing your basic eating plan, you may need to supplement. Supplements can often provide the additional nutrition you require without overwhelming your internal operating systems with excess calories and sheer volume.

Because individual requirements vary so widely, it's almost impossible for me (or any expert) to specify what supplements you might need. I can and will offer you some general recommendations, but for an accurate assessment of your nutritional deficiencies and imbalances, visit a health professional qualified to provide you with a complete nutritional profile. Blood and urine tests can pinpoint dietary defects that may be interfering with the efficient operation of your internal processes.

The list that follows includes some of the more useful supplements widely available. Note that several of these are compound substances. Because nutrients work together in the body, combining a number of compatible supplements often enhances their effectiveness. (The observation that the whole is greater than the sum of its parts applies here.) Whenever you use nutritional additives, always consult the label for proper dosage and consumption schedule information.

Vitamins

Essential to the growth, maintenance, and repair of the body, vitamins play a vital role in all metabolic functions. Unless a specific severe deficiency is diagnosed, vitamins are best taken in combination. (An excessive quantity of a single vitamin often triggers harmful biochemical reactions and imbalances.)

The most valuable multiple vitamin compounds usually include:

B Complex. Without B vitamins, carbohydrates, proteins, and fats can't be converted into energy that the body can use. B vitamins are essential to nervous system maintenance. They also help sustain the integrity of intestinal tract muscles and enhance liver functions.

Vitamin C. This vitamin is a powerful antioxidant. It's also essential for the development and maintenance of connective tissue in skin, ligaments, and bones. Vitamin C assists in the formation of red blood cells and the scar tissue needed to accelerate the healing of wounds.

Vitamin E. This vitamin is also an antioxidant. Vitamin E nourishes cells and promotes muscle growth. It protects the body from pollutants and poisons created by the breakdown of organic substances, and is essential to the digestive system and the production of certain hormones.

Antioxidants

Free radicals are nasty toxic substances that invade the body and damage cells. Antioxidants are free-radical scavengers. If antioxidants aren't present to hunt down and eliminate free radicals, normal cellular deterioration is accelerated, causing our internal infrastructure to age faster. Antioxidants also improve protein synthesis and tissue regeneration after exercise. Most antioxidant supplements now available include combinations of vitamins A, C, and E, beta-carotene, selenium, zinc, and other effective free-radical fighters. See also Green Tea under Herbs (page 57)

Enzymes

Enzymes govern all the body's chemical reactions. Some enzymes dissolve food so that it can be absorbed through the intestinal walls. Deep within our internal fuel management systems, other enzymes help convert nutrients into functional construction materials. Because most foods are low in enzymatic activity, enzyme supplements can often assist metabolic activity significantly.

There are specific enzymes best equipped to aid in the digestion of different food classes. If you're shopping for an enzyme supplement, be sure to choose one that includes all the enzymes you'll need to process all your food. Look for what I call the "Four Aces"—cellulase, for fiber; lipase, for fat; amylase, for carbs; and protease, for proteins.

DHEA is a prevalent hormone in the body that declines with age. It is now available over the counter, without a prescription. Experts claim that

DHEA supplementation can reset your internal biological clock making you feel and look younger. DHEA's effects make it a useful supplement for active people that can also rev up a sluggish sex drive. **But please check with your doctor for personalized administration of DHEA.**

Minerals

Minerals play a role in every function of the human body. Simply put, without minerals we cannot live a normal healthy life. Unfortunately, many of the foods we consume are deficient in minerals; therefore supplementation is necessary. Since minerals are difficult for the body to ingest, the best way to obtain minerals is through liquid or capsules. A multimineral product is your best choice.

Chromium, often called insulin's "essential co-factor," helps the body manage blood sugar levels. A chromium deficiency can intensify sugar cravings, increase blood fat levels, and slow metabolic rates. Some scientists link chromium deficiencies to heart problems and diabetes. Chromium occurs naturally in food but is often lost in processing and refining. The U.S. Department of Agriculture recently reported that about 85 percent of us aren't getting enough chromium in our diets.

Lactobacillus Acidophilus

We need a fully functional intestinal tract to effectively assimilate the nutrients present in the foods we eat. Lactobacillus acidophilus (LA) helps maintain intestinal integrity by keeping the toxins that populate the digestive tract under control. If you're afflicted with digestive problems and/or bowel irregularities, LA, highly recommended by health professionals around the world, may help. The best way to obtain LA is by consuming natural yogurt.

L-Carnitine

Despite our best efforts, without enough of the lipotropic agent L-Carnitine (L-C) in our systems, we may experience slow progress in our fat reduction attempts. L-C is an amino acid compound that helps the body burn fat by shuttling it into tissues where it can be used for fuel. L-C may have a beneficial effect on the heart, and some research indicates that L-C may increase overall energy levels.

Melatonin

The hormone melatonin is known to stimulate the production of other hormones in the body, especially human growth hormone and the insulin-like growth factor-1 (IGF-1). These hormones help the body maintain lean muscle, increase metabolic rates, and stimulate energy production. Melatonin is also an effective insomnia treatment.

Protein

The eating plan I'm recommending should deliver all the protein your body needs. If it doesn't or if you can't find enough lean protein sources that you actually like to eat, there are a number of excellent protein supplements widely available. Choose one that provides all the essential amino acids: isoleucine, lysine, phenylalanine, tryptophan, histidine, leucine, methionine, cysteine, threonine, and valine.

Protein supplements are available in powders, tablets, capsules, snack bars, and chewable wafers.

L-Arginine has recently become a popular supplement with its sexual mimicking effects similar to the synthetic Viagra. L-Arginine has the ability to increase the levels of nitric oxide in the body, which is responsible for forcing blood into a man's penis, thus stimulating erections. In women, although not as well documented, nitric oxide increases blood flow to the clitoris, making it more sensitive. L-Arginine is an amino acid that is also known to stimulate the pituitary gland to release growth hormone.

Herbs

Herbal supplements offer a wide variety of health benefits. There is an almost infinite number of herbs and plant products that can enhance your body's appearance, performance, and general well-being. Following are brief descriptions of some of the herbals you might find helpful in your fat reduction efforts.

Ephedra (Ma huang), an herbal stimulant, has become widely recommended as a weight loss tonic. This is an extremely potent herb that increases core body temperature and acts as a diuretic. **Caution: Ephedra can cause unpleasant and sometimes dangerous side effects if overused or abused**.

Ginkgo Biloba is an excellent herb for improving the circulation of blood and oxygen to the brain. It is also known to improve memory capacity and treat depression, and is used quite effectively for psychological impotency.

Ginseng provides some benefit to almost all body functions, including the cardiovascular system. This herb boosts athletic performance and is often helpful in fighting mental and physical fatigue and stress. It also is regarded as a sexual tonic.

Gotu Kola and *Guarana* are two popular herbs commonly used in fat reduction formulas for their stimulating effects on the central nervous system. When consumed conservatively, both these herbs are safe and effective, while they both provide other benefits to the body and brain.

Green Tea is a potent antioxidant and fat-burning herb that stimulates a sluggish metabolism and provides a variety of health benefits. Sipping hot green tea in place of coffee is a wise substitute and a lot better for you, too. But don't sip it at night as it can cause insomnia.

Kelp is used in many weight management programs to help stimulate metabolic rates. Kelp is rich in minerals—especially iodine, a substance essential for thyroid health. This herb also assists operational functions of the kidneys, heart, and muscular system.

Licorice can be an aid in the production of hormones that diminish the harmful effects of stress and fatigue. It's also a mild laxative and a cleansing agent for the bloodstream.

Fuel Management Techniques

To help you increase the effectiveness of your fat-burning eating plan, I've gathered some helpful hints and useful suggestions from a variety of sources:

▶ Broil meats, poultry, and fish instead of frying or baking.

▶ Use real butter in place of synthetic substitutes.

▶ Prefer whole grain bread to those limp processed white bread pretenders.

▶ When using commercially prepared and processed foods, try to avoid glutamates, and other additives you're not familiar with.

▶ Don't overcook vegetables. Vitamins and enzymes will be lost. The fresher vegetables smell, the more nutritious they'll be.

▶ Don't peel apples, cucumbers, potatoes, zucchini, etc. The skin is loaded with nutritional fiber, which is good for your digestive tract.

▶ Trim all excess fat from beef.

▶ Buy kosher hot dogs and bologna. They're made from beef and generally are less fatty than nonkosher products. They also don't contain mysterious additives.

▶ Enjoy your meals, and eat slowly. Chew your food thoroughly. Give your digestive system time to do its work.

▶ Include avocados, peanut butter, olives, nuts, and extra-virgin olive oil in your eating plan. The fats and oils in these foods raise HDL (good cholesterol) levels and promote muscle growth.

▶ Don't deny yourself any food you really like. Adjust your fuel mix to make room for these necessary pleasures—but remember to stay balanced.

▶ If you think missing meals will accelerate fat loss, think again. Skipping meals throws your internal operating systems into a crisis mode. Glandular control centers shut down your normal energy management protocols, forcing your body to use muscle as fuel—not fat.

▶ Drink lots of water. Water helps regulate your body temperature, speeds delivery of oxygen to tissues, assists in the kidneys' waste removal efforts, enhances muscle growth, and aids in the fat-burning process.

4

Permanently Boosting Metabolism

The TV sitcom *Home Improvement* chronicled the misadventures of Tim "The Tool Man" Taylor, an affable wacko who made his living hosting a television show for do-it-yourself buffs. A typical exchange between The Tool Man and his sidekick, a straitlaced old-fashioned hardware store guy named Al, would go something like this:

Tim: Whatcha got there, Al?

Al: Well, Tim, it's something new—the most advanced, most efficient lawn tractor ever manufactured.

Tim: Really? Let's give it a try.
(Then The Tool Man would fire up the tractor, chop some furniture to bits, and slice the toes off a couple of audience members.)

Al: So how'd you like it?

Tim: Not bad. But you know what? It needs more power. *Grrr.* (Tim always growled when he said, heard, or even thought about the phrase "more power.")

Al: Well, gee, Tim, it has a state-of-the-art titanium Z-46 maxi-blaster.

Tim: Yeah, but if we could hook this baby up to a modified NASCAR turbo . . .

So it went every week. The Tool Man would discover another weed whacker or leaf blower or chain saw that, with just a few adjustments, could be made faster, louder, meaner, and, of course, more powerful. And

Tim would make whatever harebrained modifications he thought would accomplish that demented mission. And the results, sadly, were always the same: abject, painful failure. Houses blew up; pets caught fire; ambulances were called; arrests were made.

Okay, The Tool Man was an idiot, but that doesn't mean we shouldn't respect and admire his insatiable appetite for improvement and innovation. The man was a visionary, a dreamer, a backyard scientist. Only his incredible incompetence denied him the success he sought.

Like Tim Taylor we are going to take a well-designed, perfectly functional machine and try to make it more efficient and, yes, more powerful. Unlike the hapless Tool Man, however, we will succeed, because we'll actually know what we're doing.

The human body is a fantastic machine with a huge capacity for restoration, renovation, and replenishment. We'll rely on exercise and well-established body science to gain control of our machine's intricate fuel management systems and set in motion a series of chain reactions that, within thirty days, will tune and turbocharge our internal processes to burn fat quickly and safely.

Let's begin with a radically simplified survey of the mechanisms we'll access and the methods we'll use to tinker with their operations.

Our Muscles

All physical activity, from the blinking of an eye to digestion, salsa dancing, and the beating of your heart, is powered by muscles. There are over six hundred muscles in the human body, each consisting of bundles of tightly interlocking fibers varying in length from a couple of millimeters (the muscles that move the eyebrows) to several inches (the buttock muscles—yes, Virginia, there are muscles back there). Muscles almost always work in coordinated groups: The contraction of one muscle necessitates the relaxation of another.

To have any chance of success, your fuel reduction efforts must rely heavily on your muscles. Exercise that stimulates muscle growth and development is your most direct access to meaningful improvement of your body's fat-burning capabilities. Certain kinds of physical activity traumatize muscle cells in a good way. The biochemical stress I'm talking about actually tears relatively inert cellular elements into unstable, extremely active substances. Internal reparation abilities use physiochemical components we obtain from food to regenerate and rebuild muscle tissue. Consistent ignition of this rebuilding cycle makes muscle stronger, denser, and more chemically active—and, most important for our purposes, increases muscle cell incineration of stored fat.

When the trillions of muscle cells in our bodies are aroused, they become microscopic blast furnaces, torching fat and sugar to fuel their reconstruction activities. It has been shown that exercise which targets muscle development increases the size and power of muscle cells as well as the fat-burning efficiency of each cell. It's a wonderful thing. With the appropriate exercise strategy, you can boost fat reduction exponentially. (Don't worry, the exercise plan I'll propose won't require you to pump iron until your arms fall off.)

Our Metabolism

Body scientists use the term *metabolism* to describe the aggregate of all the intricate physical, chemical, and electrical processes constantly taking place in the body at the cellular level. The energy required to perform the thousands of metabolic functions that make up the body's twenty-four-hour-long workday is extracted from the food we consume. This energy intake is measured in thermal units called *calories*. All of our cellular systems use these calories for fuel nourishment, growth, maintenance, oxygenation, and other life-sustaining activities. Calories not needed for fuel are usually stored as fat if they are not eliminated.

Your exercise plan obviously needs to generate enough metabolic activity to burn not only the calories you're consuming every day but also the stored fat that is stubbornly tucked inside your system now. This isn't as daunting as it seems, because if you design your exercise strategy intelligently, you can expect your body's help.

Among the metabolic functions you'll find most useful as allies are *anabolism* and *catabolism*. Anabolism refers to the process through which microscopic food particles are used to construct protoplasm. The physiochemical essence of living matter, protoplasm is a gluelike, granular, grayish, and translucent substance. Protoplasm is the primary core of your body's living cells. Catabolism is the process that reduces protoplasm to its simpler, more unstable components.

Exercise that increases the size, strength, or work capacity of body cells provokes a catabolic/anabolic cycle that burns calories. If we exercise regularly and wisely, we increase not only the amount of this fuel consumption but the burn rate as well.

Our Cardiovascular System

While the body fat we see overflowing our waistlines or padding our butts may seem to be the primary target of our fat reduction offensives, many of us should also be more concerned about some thick greasy deposits we can't see: fat buildup within our arteries.

The arterial walls of a healthy infant are smooth, clean, strong, and elastic. Thanks to a national diet too rich in sugars, animal fats, and lard, the arteries of the average American adult are marbled with toxic residue. Over time, the fatty deposits we begin accumulating the day we discover fast food harden into troublesome obstructions. The end result can be high blood pressure, blood clots, arteriosclerosis, or one of several other dangerous disorders.

Luckily, the exercise strategy we'll use to power our fat reduction efforts will also produce substantial improvements in our arterial network. A regular schedule of physical activity will impose healthy demands on your heart, simulating an acceleration of blood flow and increasing its volume and oxygenation. As you exercise, your heart performs like an open faucet, pumping large quantities of swiftly moving blood through your circulatory pathways and scrubbing the inner walls of your arteries.

As you strengthen your heart with exercise (it is a muscle, after all), another benefit is realized: reduced wear and tear on your body's fuel pump. A well-conditioned heart can perform its vital functions at a steady, comfortable pace because each heartbeat produces enough force to move large volumes of blood through the body. A weak heart needs to beat much more often to process the same workload.

A normal heart rate is about 72 beats per minute (bpm). If you establish and sustain a reasonable exercise habit, you can expect to reduce that rate to around 60 bpm. If we do the math, we find that a reconditioned cardiovascular system can save 720 heartbeats an hour, 17,280 a day, and well over 6 million beats per year. You needn't be a cardiologist to recognize that saving 60 million heartbeats a decade is an excellent way to avoid the coronary wear and tear that hospitalizes or kills so many Americans.

Ladies and Gentlemen, Start Your Engines

Early in my career, almost thirty years ago, the relative value of various exercise regimens was frequently debated. On one side of the controversy, the aerobics crowd trumpeted the benefits of slow, steady regimens that featured jogging, fitness walking, and aerobic dancing. You will live longer, these zealots promised, with a stronger heart and more powerful lungs. You won't overexert yourself, and you'll lose weight, too. "Whatever," the anti-aerobic bodybuilders sneered. Fitness is more than cardiovascular health. What about strength? Power? Muscle definition?

Fortunately for me (and for you), I never limited myself or the athletes I trained to a single rigid approach. I've always been open to investigation and experimentation. As time passed, I worked my way through hundreds of studies and theories and hypotheses.

What I found is that a carefully designed, fully integrated exercise strategy that offers variety is the fastest, most effective path to accelerated fat reduction and improved health!

Aerobic Exercise

Any activity that raises your heart rate to between 65 and 85 percent of its maximum level for an extended period of time is considered an aerobic exercise. Typically, you need to move at a steady (though not necessarily uncomfortable) pace for a minimum of twenty to thirty minutes to reach and maintain this level of exertion. Until its corrosive impact on joints became well known, jogging and other high-impact activities were the most popular aerobic exercises. Today, many aerobic workouts involve the use of stationary bikes, treadmills, stair climbers, elliptical steppers, or scores of other fitness machines. Although there are wildly varying levels of intensity and benefit, almost anything you can do for an extended period of time has some aerobic value. Power walking, dancing, swimming, roller-skating, and dozens of other activities can be used to provide your body with the benefits of aerobic exercise.

And those benefits are substantial. Aerobic training will strengthen your heart and cardiovascular system, and improve respiratory efficiency. Regular sustained aerobic activity will reduce blood sugar levels, lower blood pressure, improve fat utilization levels, raise HDL (good cholesterol), and lower LDL (bad cholesterol).

And, yes, burn fat.

Eventually.

If you like the relatively gentle strain and easy pace of aerobic exercise and have about an hour you can set aside four days a week, aerobics may indeed be the way to go. You'll lose fat slowly, but you will lose it.

To fuel your aerobic activities, your body will first draw upon circulating blood sugars and carbohydrate stores. When these energy sources are depleted, the body shifts to a blend of oxygen and fat to fuel itself. How quickly you reach the fat-burning phase depends on the sugars and carbs available and the intensity and duration of your aerobic workout. Marathon runners "carbo-load" the night before the big race to delay the depletion of oxygen and fat reserves as long as possible. Because you want the fat-burning phase of your aerobics to kick in as quickly as possible, you'll want to keep carb consumption low to realize the maximum benefits available from your workout.

Generally speaking, only about 40 percent of the time spent in conventional aerobic exercise converts fat to fuel. If you want faster, more dramatic fat loss, you have to move beyond aerobics to activities that offer a higher return on your exercise investment.

Aerobic Exercise Fuel Consumption

Blood Sugar | Fat
Workout Period [30–60 Minutes/Typical]

Fat
Post-Workout Period [2–12 Hours/Typical]

Anaerobic Exercise Fuel Consumption

Blood Sugar | Fat
Workout Period [20–45 Minutes/Typical]

Fat
Post-Workout Period [1–2 Days/Typical]

AEROBIC: During the first 50–70 percent of most aerobic sessions, blood sugar is the primary fuel source. Since aerobic workouts typically do not traumatize muscle tissues, the post-workout metabolism, or fat-burning operations, have less caloric demands as compared with anaerobic workouts. To accelerate fat burning during aerobic activity, it is best to perform these workouts on an empty stomach to deplete blood sugar levels sooner, forcing the body to shift to burning fat.

ANAEROBIC: During typical anaerobic workouts sugar—that is, blood sugar and glycogen—are the primary fuel sources. Fat isn't called into action until later on in an anaerobic session. However, due to the tissue-traumatizing effect of anaerobic exercise, the post-workout metabolism has enormous caloric, or fat-burning demands. Therefore, the goal during these workouts is to focus on developing the muscles; then the body will automatically switch to a fat-burning mode afterward to recuperate its traumatized tissues, also called anabolism!

The Integrated Approach

While the body's need for aerobic stimulation can't be disputed, there are better and faster ways to burn fat. A wealth of scientific data indicates that traditional low- to moderate-intensity aerobic exercise burns fat primarily during the workout. Most aerobics do little to stimulate your post-workout metabolic rate, at least for any extended period of time.

You know from experience that your car burns more fuel in stop-and-go city driving than it does cruising the interstate. Your body, although much more cleverly designed than any automobile, ultimately burns more fat as the result of "short-burst" exercise than it does in fueling slower, steadier activities.

Which brings us to the value of *anaerobic* exercise.

Anaerobic activity is any powerful burst of hard, quick physical action that drastically quickens your heart rate and leaves you gasping for air. Weight training (using free weights or various machines or the resistance your own body can provide) is the most commonly recognized example of anaerobic exercise. Almost any aerobic activity can become anaerobic if it becomes intense enough. Jogging along the beach is aerobic; sprinting home with the neighbor's pit bull in hot pursuit is anaerobic. Strolling through a nature preserve is aerobic; hiking from the floor of the Grand Canyon to its rim is extremely anaerobic. Cycling along the lakefront is aerobic; trying to catch the leader in the Tour de France in the Pyrenees is anaerobic. Gliding around the ice rink on a Sunday afternoon is aerobic; Olympic speed skating is anaerobic.

To fuel anaerobic activities, your body relies on its most accessible, fastest-burning energy sources: carbohydrates (which include sugars). When it exhausts its carb reserves, the body has no choice but to shift to burning fat for energy.

I know. This is good. This is what we want.

Too bad our bodies won't allow it.

The catch is, few of us can maintain an anaerobic heart rate (90–100 percent of the heart's maximum work capacity) for very long. While millions of joggers can shuffle along for hours, even world-class sprinters can't sustain their anaerobic activity of choice for much more than forty seconds.

To take advantage of the body's fuel management system without killing anyone I'm going to suggest an exercise plan based on a concept I call Variable Intensity Training. VIT makes your body's fuel-burning and energy usage protocols powerful allies in your war on fat.

Unlike the long, slow, steady pace common in traditional aerobic workouts, VIT requires you to move into and out of both aerobic and anaerobic ranges. Short, explosive bursts of activity alternate with periods of moderate exertion.

A jogger who wants to utilize VIT principles might design a workout that would look something like this:

▶ a five-minute steady pace warm-up leading to . . .
▶ a thirty-second sprint followed by . . .
▶ thirty seconds of brisk walking or light jogging followed by . . .
▶ eight to twelve repetitions of the same go-hard, go-easy cycle and . . .
▶ a five-minute cooldown.

By using my VIT approach our anonymous jogger has dramatically increased the fat-burning value of his thirty-minute workout by 20–30 percent (compared to the fat burned with sixty minutes of steady jogging).

VIT can be applied to any exercise option—walking, jogging, running, biking, dancing, stair stepping, treadmilling, rowing, whatever. Do whatever you enjoy doing, but frequently during the course of your workout do it harder and faster. Many aerobic training machines give you computerized control of intensity levels, making VIT principles extremely easy to execute. As you become acclimated to the VIT approach, you'll find yourself able to manage more frequent bursts of anaerobic effort.

The Afterburn Bonus

In addition to allowing you to burn between 20–30 percent more fat per hour during your workouts, VIT has another even more exciting benefit: ***Because of the way your metabolism reacts to VIT activity, you'll continue burning fat long after your exercise sessions have ended.*** To understand why that is, we'll make a brief visit to the fascinating world of muscle fibers.

If you've ever watched a track meet, you may have noticed that not all track and field athletes look alike. A distance runner's body is thin, with long, fluid muscles. The sprinters are bigger, with denser, more highly defined bodies. The shot-putters and discus throwers are just plain huge all over.

All these athletes are fit; the differences in their bodies are a reflection of the training they used to excel in their respective specialties. Each competitor concentrated on a specific type of muscle fiber in his or her conditioning activities.

The long-distance runners trained primarily slow twitch (ST) muscle fibers. These relatively lengthy elastic fibers are slow, steady, contractors. The body recruits these fibers for steady long-haul activities. (If you want, think of them as having kind of an Energizer Bunny quality.)

The long-distance runner typically has developed more ST muscle fibers than the sprinter. To excel at her specialty, the sprinter needs an abundance of fast twitch (FT) muscle fibers. The FT fibers that the sprinter uses for the explosive powerful bursts she needs to propel herself down the track are shorter, stronger, and more explosive than the ST muscle fibers the long-distance runner favors. (In a cartoon world, the Road Runner would play the FT muscle fiber.) The shot put and discus athletes have pumped and bulked and grown their FT muscle fibers to the extent that yields cannon-like results.

By everyday standards all these athletes are in excellent shape. The connection between them and your use of VIT principles in your fat reduction efforts can be seen in the differences in their training programs. Let's use some principles of each training program to add variety and benefits to your VIT.

The primary training goal of the three-miler was, no doubt, optimum cardiovascular capacity and stamina. Long (I mean really long) runs were the centerpiece of his workouts. The sprinter trained for raw speed at short distances by using interval principles primarily, with some weight lifting sessions. The shot-putter's regimen was probably based almost exclusively on resistance training.

Because she is not like normal humans, the long-distance runner's aerobically rich ST training may have burned more calories each training day than did your typical fitness fanatic in aerobics class. But the fat-burning benefits of the sprinter's or the shot-putter's workout were more productive, despite less ground being covered, with a large number of rest intervals integrated within the workout.

Ah, but let's take a look at what happened whenever these athletes took a day off.

Deep within the muscle cells of the long-distance runner, a reaction different from the explosive counterpart occurred. Several hours after she had finished, much of the fat burning that was going to occur had occurred. The resilient, placid ST muscle fibers she'd abused all day had pretty much restored themselves.

Within the cellular structures of the sprinter and the shot-putter, on the other hand, a serious and massive reconstruction project was under way. The repeated demand for intense explosive activity had created microscopic tears to millions of lean tissue fibers. Repair and regeneration would take at least a day, maybe two or longer. The metabolic processes charged with completing these repairs worked well into the night and possibly for days to follow. Where did the recuperation energy for all this intracellular labor come from?

From the sugar and fat stored inside the athletes' bodies. And, of course, the energy was burned—all day and all night until the muscle cells were completely restored. (And while they were at it, this biochemical construction crew used whatever protein was handy to increase the strength and size of the new muscle cells.)

Yes, it's true, anaerobic exercise of any kind increases both the efficiency and duration of the metabolic processes that burn fat. Use VIT principles in your exercise plan, and you, too, can burn body fat while you sleep. (See the chart on page 71.)

The No-Excuses Workout

I'm guessing that just about now you've absorbed all you need to absorb about exercise approaches and metabolism, and the interaction between them. I suspect that practical questions are pushing their way into your frontal lobe.

Questions such as:

▶ Do I have to lift weights?
▶ Do I have to buy one of those giant fitness machines?
▶ Do I have to sprint? I haven't sprinted since I was twelve. Really, do I have to sprint?
▶ Do I have to join a health club or a gym or whatever they call them now?
▶ It gets cold up here. Do I have to go out in the cold every day?
▶ I'm really busy. When will I find time to exercise?
▶ Do I have to wear Lycra?

No. No. No. No. No. You won't need as much time as you think. And no.

At the beginning of our time together I promised to deliver a fat-burning process that normal, average, everyday people could use to reach reasonable health and fitness goals. Well, I'm going to do just that. I think you agree that my eating recommendations are simple, sensible, and easy to accept. I believe you'll find the exercise part of the regimen equally tolerable.

What I want from you is seven minutes a day. But not every day, maybe three or four days per week. That's it.

The seven-minute routine I've developed for you can be done **anytime, anywhere.** This is my No-Excuses Workout (NEW), which requires no special equipment. The NEW includes both aerobic and anaerobic components that incorporate resistance exercises and cardiovascular conditioning. It's a total body workout, engaging all your major muscle groups. Make the NEW a weekly habit, and you can expect metabolic rate enhancement, respiratory improvement, and noticeable increases in coordination, flexibility, stamina, and endurance.

A detailed description of the exercises included in your NEW follows, along with photos (by Jim Amentler) illustrating each exercise.

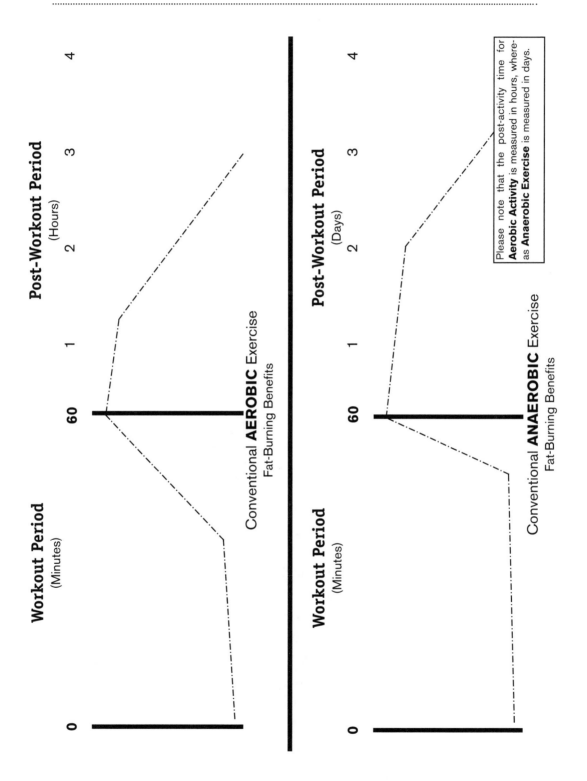

Please note that the post-activity time for **Aerobic Activity** is measured in hours, whereas **Anaerobic Exercise** is measured in days.

John Abdo's "No-Excuses Workout"
NEW
This workout can be performed anywhere and anytime.
No equipment is necessary.

Features and Benefits

Cardiovascular conditioning   Body shaping

Flexibility improvement   Fat burner

Muscle strengthening   Endurance

Metabolic booster   *and more!*

Rules

▶ Do not eat 1 hour before workout.

▶ Eat a healthy meal within 60 minutes after workout.

Exercise Instructions

1. *March.* Stand up with your fists clenched and your arms bent at the elbow. Begin to pump your arms and legs simultaneously in a marching motion. Imagine that you're the grand marshal of the Rose Bowl parade. March as fast as you can, pumping your arms and legs as high as they'll go, for 30 seconds.

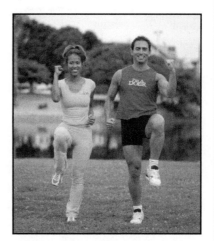

2. *Push-up.* Lie facedown and place your hands next to your chest. Push your body upward until your arms become straight at the elbows. Keep your knees on the floor if you can't

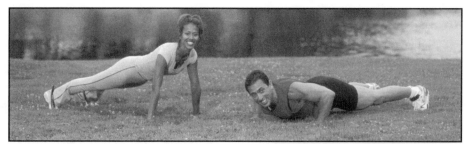

complete a full push-up as seen in the photo. Do as many push-ups as you can in 30 seconds.

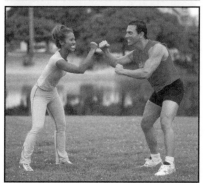

3. *Squat.* Stand with your feet directly below your shoulders or slightly wider. Keeping your back straight, slowly bend your knees until your thighs are parallel with the floor. Use a chair as a balance aid if necessary. Repeat the squats for 30 seconds.

4. *Shadow Box.* Assume a comfortable balanced stance. Clench your fists and punch the air in front of you, left-right, left-right, etc. Rotate your torso slightly and pivot with each punch. Don't overextend your arms or snap your elbows. Continue for 30 seconds.

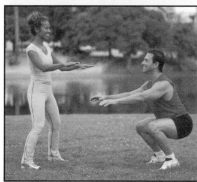

5. *V Sits.* Sit at the edge of a chair or bench. Lean back. Slowly lift your knees upward as high as you can. Squeeze your abdominal and hip muscles as you lift your knees. Slowly return your feet to the floor. Repeat for 30 seconds.

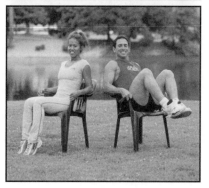

6. *Leg Raise.* Stand upright and hold onto a chair or broomstick with one hand for balance. Keeping your left leg straight, slowly raise your right leg in front of you as high as possible. Slowly swing your right leg as far back as it will go, then kick it forward to begin again. Swing your right leg in a front-to-back pendulum motion for 30 seconds.

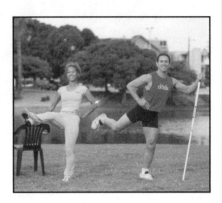

7. *Leg Raise.* Repeat exercise 6 using your left leg.

8. *Calf Raise.* Stand upright, feet directly below your shoulders. If necessary, use a chair or broomstick to maintain balance. Keeping your toes on the floor, raise your heels as high as you can, bending only at the ankles. Repeat rapidly for 30 seconds.

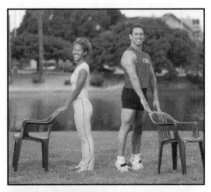

9. *Jumping Jacks.* Just as you did back in high school gym class, start with your feet together and your arms at your sides. Jump (not too high), and as you jump, spread your legs and try to join your hands over your head. Return to the starting position. Keep this up for 30 seconds.

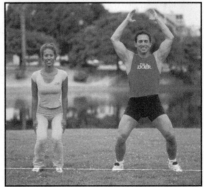

10. ***Crunch.*** Lie on your back with both knees bent and your feet flat on the floor. Place your hands on your stomach. Lift your head and chest until you feel your abdominal muscles tighten. Return your upper body to the floor. Repeat as often as you can for 30 seconds.

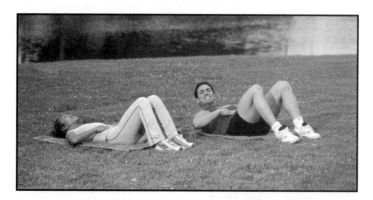

11. ***Swim Strokes.*** Resurrecting an obscure dance move from the sixties, you do the "crawl" forward for 15 seconds, and then the backstroke for 15 more. Rotate your arms in wide circles, reaching and pivoting your torso just as you would in the pool.

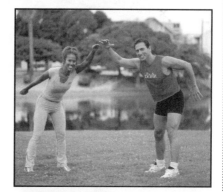

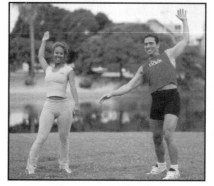

12. **Leg Kicks.** Sit on a chair or bench. Lean back and proceed as if trying to kick your shoes off. Right foot first, then the left. Alternate legs for 30 seconds.

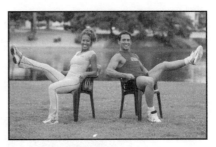

13. **Toe Touch/Overhead Reach.** Stand up or sit in a chair. Lean forward and try to touch your toes. Don't force it; go only as far as you can. Maintain your balance by keeping your feet flat on the floor, and be aware of your body position at all times. After reaching down as far as you can, reach up as far as you can. Repeat for 30 seconds.

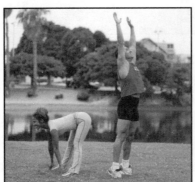
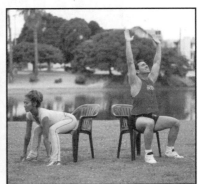

14. **Crossover Toe Touch.** Stand upright, feet directly below your shoulders. Spread your arms out to each side. Bend forward and at the same time twist your torso to bring your right hand down toward your left foot. Return to your upright starting position. Bend forward again, this time to bring your left hand down toward your right foot. Repeat for 30 seconds.

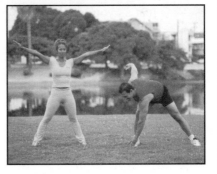

Application

Perform each movement for 30 seconds then move onto the next. If you cannot make 30 seconds, then perform as many repetitions as you can for each exercise within the 30 seconds, and then move on.

Once a full circuit is completed, take a 1–2 minute rest, and then repeat if you can.

▶ Read the Doer Oath before every workout (page 176).
▶ Recite affirmations during your sessions.
▶ Breathe normally.
▶ Stretch as often as you can.
▶ Drink plenty of water.
▶ Listen to music that makes you feel energetic.
▶ Don't listen to the news or watch TV.
▶ Feel your body, touch it everywhere, and talk to it.

Beginner	1 Circuit	=	7 minutes
Intermediate	2 Circuits	=	14 minutes, with one 2-minute rest period
Advanced	3 Circuits	=	21 minutes, with two 2-minute rest periods
Ultra Advanced	4 Circuits	=	28 minutes, with three 2-minute rest periods

Frequency

Beginner	Every other day, or 3–4 times weekly
Intermediate	Every other day, or 3–4 times weekly
Advanced	Two days on and one day off in succession
Ultra Advanced	Two days on and one day off in succession

The No-Excuses Workout Time-Code

Time	Exercises
0:00–0:30	March
0:30–1:00	Push-up
1:00–1:30	Squat
1:30–2:00	Shadow Box
2:00–2:30	V-Sits
2:30–3:00	Leg Raise [front/back; right leg]
3:00–3:30	Leg Raise [front/back; left leg]
3:30–4:00	Calf Raise
4:00–4:30	Jumping Jacks
4:30–5:00	Crunch
5:00–5:30	Swim Strokes [front/back]
5:30–6:00	Leg Kicks
6:00–6:30	Toe Touch/Overhead Reach [seated or standing]
6:30–7:00	Crossover Toe Touch
7:00–9:00	Rest Period: May Repeat Circuit

There are only a couple of guidelines to keep in mind.

Perform each exercise for thirty seconds. If you can't continue steadily for the thirty seconds, complete as many repetitions as you can. If something hurts, stop. Return to the exercise descriptions and photos to verify that you're doing the exercise correctly.* Don't watch television or listen to talk radio while exercising. Music is great, but not if it's distracting or puts you to sleep.

Consult your physician before attempting this routine if you failed the stress test in Chapter 2, if you suffer from heart trouble or high blood pressure, or if you are clinically obese. If you are significantly overweight or unusually shaped, you may find some of the NEW movements difficult to complete exactly as described. Without pushing, try to complete as much of each movement as you can. Exercising consistently, you'll be amazed that you'll be able to do a little better each day.

Initially, you should complete only one circuit of exercises per session and limit yourself to no more than three or four sessions each week. Ideally, your NEW should be performed before breakfast. A substantial body of research suggests that early workouts burn more fat than those done later in the day. If you choose to do another NEW workout, the best time for your second session is about a half hour before your Window of Opportunity Meal. When you exercise is obviously up to you, but if you're doubling up each day, try to allow at least three hours between your NEW sessions. And don't eat a heavy meal for at least one hour (two hours is better) prior to your NEW.

Begin with one NEW circuit three or four times a week or every other day. As your comfort, confidence, and conditioning improve, increase that frequency to two NEW circuits during each session, or one followed by another. When two circuits no longer present a challenge for you, increase your regimen to three or four circuits per session, or divide two circuits twice a day. Remember to rest for one to two minutes between circuits. When you reach this advanced level, stay there. Don't spend more than thirty to forty minutes per session.

*John Abdo's "No-Excuses Workout" video is a complete NEW watch-and-participate routine.

While you'll probably want to add some variety to your exercise strategies as time passes, the NEW is an excellent kick-start program. Combine your NEW with your balanced meal plan, and within thirty days you'll be amazed at the changes you have made to your body.

Optional Enhancements
Flexercise

Stiff and lethargic muscles are vulnerable to injury, and until they become loose, they are incapable of optimum performance. While you needn't achieve extraordinary flexibility to exercise competently, a properly stretched body will certainly enhance the effectiveness of your workouts and increase your enjoyment of recreational activity.

The twelve stretching exercises below are designed to improve joint mobility and ease of motion. Follow the instructions that accompany each diagram carefully. Proceed cautiously; I don't want you overexerting tissues you didn't even know you had. Stretch slowly and patiently. Don't force movement if your body protests, and don't bounce. As with any exercise you try, stop immediately if you feel pain.

Muscle and Joint Flexibility Exercises
Names and Descriptions
(Refer to Illustrations)

Number	Name

1.   Torso Twists

While standing upright with feet at a shoulders'-width stance, keep your chest up so that your back (spine) obtains a vertical upright position. Lift your arms so they become parallel with the floor and bent at the elbows. Rotate slowly to one side until you feel a stretch in your waistline and lower back, then slowly rotate your upper body in a circular

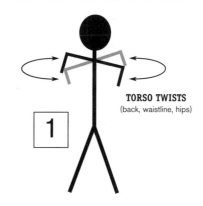

TORSO TWISTS
(back, waistline, hips)

1

fashion to the opposite side. Repeat these
twists or body circles 10–20 times.
(Perform slow and controlled.)

2.   Side Leans

While standing upright with feet at a
shoulders'-width stance, lift one arm overhead while keeping the other arm at your
side. Lean to the side of the lowered arm to
feel a stretching effect, but make sure both
feet stay in contact with the floor. After
leaning and holding for about 2–3 seconds,
slowly reverse to the other side: lower the
overhead arm and lift the lowered arm.
Repeat this on both sides 3–5 times.

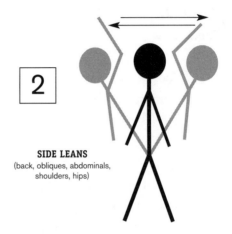

SIDE LEANS
(back, obliques, abdominals,
shoulders, hips)

3.   Squat

While standing upright with feet set slightly
wider than shoulders' width, grasp a firm
object for balance. Slowly squat or lower your
hips, trying to keep your feet flat on the
ground. Lower yourself as low as you can and
then raise yourself up in a slow but controlled
fashion. Repeat 3–5 times. (Do not bounce or
fall into the squat.)

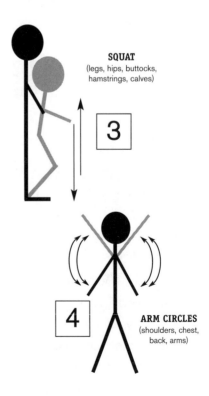

SQUAT
(legs, hips, buttocks,
hamstrings, calves)

4.   Arm Circles

While standing, lock the elbows of both arms
and then slowly start to rotate your arms to
make circles with them. Perform 5 to 10 with
the arms in one direction, and then 5 to 10 in
the other direction. Perform slowly and with
control.

ARM CIRCLES
(shoulders, chest,
back, arms)

5.   Forward Leans (Standing)

While standing upright with feet at a shoulders'-width stance, hang your arms in front of your body and then slowly lean forward, reaching down with your hands. Lean as far forward as your back muscles will permit, then hold that position for 3–5 seconds. Slowly return to an upright position. Repeat 2–3 times. (Do not bounce.)

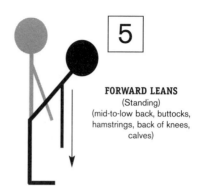

FORWARD LEANS
(Standing)
(mid-to-low back, buttocks, hamstrings, back of knees, calves)

6.   Forward Leans (Seated)

While seated upright, place your feet flat on the floor at shoulders' width. Lower your chest to your knees while reaching with your hands toward the floor. Lean as far forward as your back muscles will permit, then hold that position for 3–5 seconds. Slowly return to an upright position. Repeat 2–3 times. (Do not bounce.)

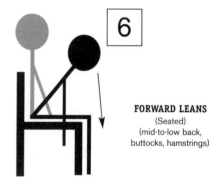

FORWARD LEANS
(Seated)
(mid-to-low back, buttocks, hamstrings)

7.   Cat Stretch

While lying on your stomach, place the palms of both hands firmly on the floor just outside your chest. Keeping your hips and thighs pressed against the floor, push yourself upward, using your chest and shoulders to arch your back rearward. Push your chest and back as high as you feel comfortable, then hold for 2–3 seconds before returning to the floor. Repeat slowly 2–3 times.

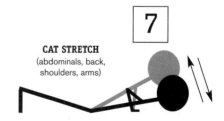

CAT STRETCH
(abdominals, back, shoulders, arms)

8.   *Pendulum*

While seated on the floor, spread your feet as far apart as you feel comfortable. Lean your torso toward one foot, trying to touch the toes of that foot with both hands. Hold this position for 2–5 seconds, then slowly rotate to the other side and try to touch the toes of that foot. Repeat each side 2–3 times slowly with no bouncing.

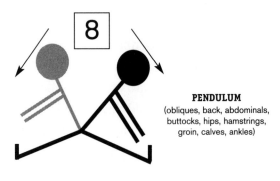

PENDULUM
(obliques, back, abdominals, buttocks, hips, hamstrings, groin, calves, ankles)

9.   *Groin Stretch*

While seated on the floor, place the bottoms of your feet together, then pull your heels close to your thighs. Holding on to your ankles, try to push your knees downward by using your elbows. You should feel a stretching sensation in the groin and thighs. Push down slowly and hold for 3–5 seconds, then let your knees up. Rest for 3–5 seconds, then repeat. Do this 2–3 times.

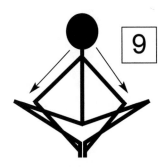

GROIN STRETCH
(groin, hips, inner thighs, knees)

10.   *Kneeling Stretch*

Place a soft mat or pillow on the floor and kneel on it. Slowly lower your buttocks to your calves until you feel a stretching sensation in the thighs, ankles, and/or knees. Hold this position for 2–3 seconds, then push yourself upward. Rest for 2–3 seconds. Repeat 2–3 times. Perform slowly with no bouncing.

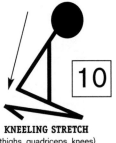

KNEELING STRETCH
(thighs, quadriceps, knees)

11.   Runner's Stretch

While standing upright, place one foot on an object about 1–2 feet off the ground. Slowly lean into that foot and hold your deepest comfortable position for 3–5 seconds, then slowly return to your starting position. Switch legs then proceed in the same fashion. Do each leg 2–3 times.

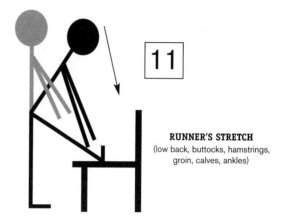

RUNNER'S STRETCH
(low back, buttocks, hamstrings, groin, calves, ankles)

12.   Ankle Stretch

While standing upright, face a wall approximately 3 feet away. Put both hands firmly against the wall and lean toward it, keeping your feet and heels flat on the floor. You will feel a stretching sensation in your ankles and calves. Hold your deepest comfortable position for 3–5 seconds, then return to the upright standing position. Rest for 2–3 seconds. Repeat 2–5 times.

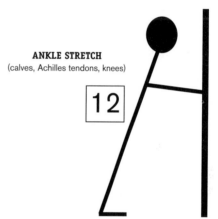

ANKLE STRETCH
(calves, Achilles tendons, knees)

The Extra Workout

With only a couple of minor behavioral adjustments, you can sneak some additional fat-burning activity into your daily routine.

First, when you head for the mall, the office, the racetrack, or wherever, don't spend a half hour driving around searching for the perfect parking place. Weather and crime stats permitting, always park your car in the farthest corner of the lot. And when grocery shopping, return your empty cart to the most inconvenient collection island. The short walks under these conditions will benefit you.

Unless your destination is the top of a skyscraper, shun elevators and escalators. Stair climbing is good for your heart, your legs, and your butt.

When you feel up to it, take two steps at a time for an even more productive mini-workout.

Rethink your approach to household chores and yard work. Strive to add an anaerobic element to lawn mowing, vacuuming, gardening, garage cleaning. Invest a little more energy in all your chores. Moving furniture, chopping wood, raking leaves, even taking out the garbage can all be worthwhile activities.

Don't choose the easy, lazy option for anything. Replace your afternoon candy bar with a brisk walk. Take the dog to the park or play catch with the kids. (Having children or a hyper German shepherd can be like living with a personal trainer.) Push yourself at every opportunity. If you get restless on one of your NEW "off" days, combine some light stretching with a walk or a bike ride. You'll be pleasantly surprised at how much your body will like your new habits.

Some Assembly Required

You now have all the information you need to begin work on your new body. It will be up to you, of course, to make the adjustments in your daily schedule and eating habits necessary for the success of your fat reduction efforts.

Am I asking too much? Demanding a top-to-bottom reorganization of your entire life? Requiring a cultlike devotion to some harsh inflexible doctrine?

I don't think so.

As promised, the changes I'm recommending are relatively minor. Some attention to meal planning and a few minutes of exercise every other day seem a fair price to pay for the substantial benefits you'll soon begin to realize.

As you replace excess body fat with lean tissue, you'll look and feel better with each passing day. You'll breathe easier, sleep sounder, and think more clearly. More important, the improvements you make will restore and rejuvenate your body's vital fundamental structures. You'll be healthier and stronger—from the inside out.

5

Thinking Fit

A promising young swimmer's dream of Olympic Gold can't come true unless she has spent thousands of hours in the pool. Only after a rookie linebacker has survived eight weeks of training camp is he capable of coping with the speed and violence of professional football. If F-16 pilots won't completely commit themselves to years of preparation and practice, they will never become astronauts.

None of these people is operating in a vacuum. The arduous physical training they need to get where they want to go must be completed within the context of their day-to-day lives—lives no less stressful than ours. The swimmer must deal with the same academic pressures, social confusion, and hormonal changes that her high school classmates face. The linebacker needs to make a home for himself in a strange city 1,500 miles away from his friends and family. The would-be astronauts have wives, children, and mortgages.

The challenges you'll encounter as you adjust your life to accommodate your fat reduction process are similar to those facing the swimmer, the linebacker, and the pilots. How do they maintain the physical and mental energy required to reach their fitness goals while at the same time fulfilling all their other obligations?

The same way you will.

By thinking fit.

Until sensible eating and exercise become an integral part of the fabric of your everyday life, your fat-burning efforts won't really blast into overdrive. Finding and accepting a fat loss program you can live with isn't quite enough; you actually have to start living it. And to develop and maintain the resolve necessary to do that, I'm going to show you how to adopt a fit person's outlook and attitudes. To become physically fit you'll need to strengthen your mind as well as your body. You have to think fit. More specifically, thinking fit is about sustaining motivation and managing stress.

Staying Committed

Assuming you're a normal human being, at some point in the next thirty days a part of you will be looking for reasons to abandon your fat-burning crusade. Deep inside most of us there's a spoiled, mischievous kid still running around loose. "Screw it," the little imp will whisper one morning. "You're tired. You had a tough day yesterday, with that moron boss constantly on your case. Sleep for an extra twenty minutes. And, hey, let's get some doughnuts on the way to work, and let's indulge at the pizza buffet at lunch and maybe stop tonight for beer and burgers and wings. You can get back on this fitness kick next week. It's only a few days away."

You may become impatient when you don't see the dramatic changes you were expecting soon enough.

Or you may become depressed, discouraged, or overwhelmed with self-doubt.

Whatever the source of your impulse to give up and regardless of the emotion in which it's wrapped, you must fight back. I hate to throw around sports clichés, but this one is too appropriate and too true to avoid: *Winners never quit and quitters never win.*

There are several options for renewing, maintaining, or strengthening your level of commitment. Use any or all of them.

Scare Yourself Straight

If you knew that your excess body fat would kill you within six months, what would you do? While your demise probably isn't quite that imminent, it's entirely accurate to remind yourself that excess fat can shorten your life and significantly erode the quality of the time you have remaining.

Look into the Future

Imagine what your new slimmer, fitter body will look like and what you will do with it. Then work backward from that image to where you are now. Ask yourself: "Okay, that's my future. What can I do today to get just one step closer to it?" It's essential to work in small increments. You can't renovate your body completely in a day or a week. But you can do one thing a day to advance toward your goal. Put enough small steps together for enough days, and you will see progress. Concentrate on the future you want and work in the present to do what needs to be done to get there.

Study Yourself

Rather than using the urge to quit (possibly coupled with your past failures) as evidence of your inability to change, step back and study yourself—just as a master mechanic would do to find and correct an engine problem. Reflect on your attitudes and behaviors. Find some small change you can make in your eating or exercise plans that will put you back on track. Evaluate your behavior honestly, and fix what needs fixing without feeling bad about yourself.

Establish Intermediate Goals

Partition your ultimate goal (the lean, fit body you're building) into smaller, more quickly attainable milestones—improving an assessment test score by 1–2 percent, for example, or moving from level 2 to level 3 on the NEW progression.

Reevaluate

If you find yourself bored or annoyed by elements of your fat-burning program, trace these attitudes to their source. Change the speed or intensity of your NEW sessions. Add music or books on tape to keep your mind active during workouts. Expand your meal options. Do something different.

Reward Yourself

As you progress toward your goals, use new clothes, show or game tickets, CDs, books, and other nonfood treats to reward yourself along the way.

Publicize Your Goals

Sharing your fitness goals with family, friends, and colleagues will make it more difficult for you to abandon your fat reduction efforts.

Find an Exercise Partner

Studies indicate that having a partner increases your chances of sticking with an exercise program by 65 percent.

Track Your Progress

Results-oriented people derive a great deal of satisfaction and motivation from tangible progress indicators. Keep a journal or use the charts I've provided.

Write a Mission Statement

A brief written declaration of what you're trying to accomplish and why can help keep your focus where it belongs.

Try to Set Personal Records

Completing forty-seven jumping jacks in thirty seconds isn't going to have the *Guinness Book of World Records* clamoring for your picture, but every time you do something better than you've ever done before, you pump yourself up and push yourself onward.

Talk to Yourself

You have a couple of choices here.

If you're the ultra-aggressive, ultracompetitive type, address your fat directly—with trash talk. Visualize each concentration of fat cells as a hated rival engaged in a no-holds-barred battle with you for control of your life. As you work out, taunt and berate the evil enemy that is trying to shut down your heart: "You're going down, you fat mess!" or "Burn, baby, burn!" or "I'm in control, not you!" and so on. (How loudly you express these sentiments is, of course, entirely up to you.)

If you respond favorably to positive reinforcement, you may find daily repetition of the following affirmations useful:

- I understand that I am in charge of my life. I will ultimately determine my fate.
- I am a winner. I may get knocked down from time to time, but I always get up.
- I know that what I see I can be, and what I believe, I can achieve.
- My body becomes leaner and healthier every day I do what must be done.
- I understand that change takes time. I am patient, but steadfast.
- I understand that change requires effort. I will work for what I want.

Take a Break

If you begin to feel burned out by your efforts, take a day or two off from your NEW. Go for an easy walk or bike ride instead. Accept the fact that on some days you simply won't be able to exercise as intensely as you'd like. No one's body is equally willing all the time. Pay attention when your body becomes stubborn, but use your brief hiatus to ensure that you come back fresh and determined for your next session.

Stress Management

Your natural aversion to change isn't the only obstacle you'll encounter as you attempt to weave sensible nutrition and regular physical activity into the fabric of your everyday life. Day-to-day existence in the twenty-first century is filled with stress.

Generally speaking, stress can be defined as any external stimulus that triggers negative emotions powerful enough to disrupt the body's normal operations. Emotional stress is a catalyst for a wide array of physical maladies, ranging from hives to bleeding ulcers to cardiac arrest. Recent research at the Johns Hopkins University Hospital suggests that from 75 to 90 percent of all doctor visits are prompted by stress-related symptoms.

It's nearly impossible to avoid stress completely, and, actually, a certain amount of stress keeps us alert, interested, and alive. But too much stress is toxic. Unrelenting stress eats away at the body's most important mechanisms. Immune system functions are degraded, leaving us more susceptible to infection. Cardiovascular and digestive operations are disrupted and damaged, increasing our risk levels for ulcers, heart attacks, and strokes. Endocrine functions are devastated, which leads to hormonal imbalances resulting in sexual impotency, lethargy, and muscle weakness.

When faced with extreme stress, the body instinctively reacts by preparing itself for lifesaving physical action—the well-known "fight or flight" response. The body perceives stress as a kind of red alert in which the major endocrine, circulatory, and respiratory systems are ordered to man their battle stations. The metabolism shuts down digestion to conserve energy. Blood vessels constrict to direct blood flow to major muscle groups (if there's any fighting or fleeing to be done, those big boys will bear the burden). Hormone levels change, and blood pressure rises dramatically.

(Interestingly, given our focus on fat reduction, whenever we experience high levels of anxiety, the body produces large amounts of cortisol, a hormone that aids in the storage of body fat.)

The body's response to stress was developed early in our evolutionary cycle as a necessary defense against the real dangers that awaited behind every rock. And those protective instincts are still occasionally valuable today (when we find ourselves face-to-face with a rabid wolverine or a used car salesman, for instance). More often than not, however, stress is dangerous. Paradoxically, the constant state of internal readiness triggered by too much stress wears out the very life source the prehistoric defense instinct was designed to protect.

By learning how best to insulate yourself from predatory stress, you won't simply be advancing your fat reduction efforts, you'll be arming yourself with a valuable survival skill.

The key to preventing toxic stress levels lies in developing behaviors and strategies that will enable you to reduce the stress stimuli in your life and counteract the stress you can't avoid with activities that provide balance, relaxation, and peace of mind.

Stress comes from a variety of sources—some negative (money problems; divorce; criticism by friends, colleagues, bosses; the death of someone close to us), and some positive (marriage, a job promotion, having a baby, going on a long vacation). Many of us manufacture our own stress. We fail to realize that stress can be the result of a negative emotional state (anger, resentment, frustration, anxiety, jealousy, depression), an outlook, or an attitude that we ourselves can manage.

The first step many of us need to take to reduce our stress levels is examining our values, perceptions, and expectations. Is the stress we're experiencing the result of someone else's behavior or our interpretation of that behavior? Do we expect too much of ourselves or of others? Do we plan, analyze, and think things through, or do we automatically react with anger or resentment to every challenge that comes our way? If you're feeling stressed on a regular basis, sit down and calmly determine how much of that stress you can diminish simply by communicating more effectively with yourself and others.

After realigning your worldview, you can adjust your behavior patterns to keep stress in check.

At Work

- Get organized and stay organized. Use a daily planner. Prioritize tasks. Keep your work area in order, with your tools, files, and other necessities in easy reach.
- Work on important projects when you're most productive—early if you're a morning person, later in the day if it takes you a while to warm up.
- Don't overcommit. Instead of automatically saying yes to every request that comes your way, give yourself time to decide if complying with the request is feasible or necessary or desirable. Instead of "Okay," or "You got it," try "Can I call you back? I need to check my schedule."
- Speaking of your schedule, avoid overbooking. Back-to-back meetings or work assignments can be tiring and burdensome. Build in a little downtime between commitments.
- Congratulate yourself when you succeed.
- Focus on the present. Rehashing the past or stewing in anxiety about the future can be extremely stressful. Concentrate on the work you need to do today, now.

▶ Keep your goals clear in your mind and make sure that you and your boss are on the same page. This clarity will allow you to prioritize your work with a valid sense of direction and purpose.

▶ Lighten up. Taking yourself less seriously allows you to laugh at errors, delays, glitches, and other work-related problems that might otherwise ruin your day.

▶ Get away from your desk or work site during lunch or breaks. Take a walk, sit in the sun, read a magazine. Forget about work for a while.

▶ Take a breather—literally. Set aside a couple of minutes each day for deep-breathing exercises. Sit comfortably, close your eyes, and fold your hands in your lap. Breathe in deeply, counting to ten as you do so. Hold your breath for a count of three, then breathe out slowly. Repeat three to five times. You'll feel your heart rate slow down and your neck and shoulder muscles relax. You will experience a pleasant sense of calm. Very refreshing. Very cleansing.

▶ Make sure your boss understands your workload. When faced with conflicting deadlines, it's important for your boss to be reminded that you don't have six hands and eight brains. Request clarification to determine what needs to be done when.

▶ Speak up. If problems with a superior or a coworker arise, discuss the difficulties calmly and respectfully. Leaving troublesome situations or issues unattended makes them (and the stress they spark) worse.

▶ Take time off. Schedule time off as you would any other appointment.

At Home

▶ Leave your work at the office. Enjoy your family and loved ones when you're at home.

▶ Don't keep your emotions to yourself. If something's bothering you, talk about it to your spouse, a family member, a friend, or a religious advisor. If you frequently feel completely overwhelmed or deeply depressed, see a psychologist or other mental health professional.

▶ Set aside a few minutes a day for solitude. Read, meditate, listen to music, take a long hot bath—whatever relaxes you. Learn about and practice structured relaxation techniques such as self-hypnosis, guided imagery, prayer, or yoga.

▸ Eat breakfast. Research suggests that people who eat breakfast every day tend to feel less anxious or stressed than those who skip the morning meal.

▸ Do one thing at a time. Don't try to help your kids with their homework and watch a ball game or iron the clothes at the same time.

▸ If work stress is threatening to burn you out, immerse yourself in a hobby or other activity you really like at home.

▸ Laugh. Spend time with people who amuse you. Enjoy friends and family members who make you laugh and those zany TV sitcom characters, too. Internet jokes and goofy movies will also reduce stress (watching the news before going to bed won't). Researchers have found that merely anticipating laughter can lower stress levels significantly. When there's nothing to laugh at, simply fake a laugh—it works!

▸ Set limits on social obligations. Don't want to go? Just say no.

▸ Set aside a couple of hours a week to deal with life's minor annoyances (food shopping, banking, the dry cleaners, automobile maintenance, balancing the checkbook, etc.).

▸ Sleep. Early to bed and early to rise may not make you any wealthier or wiser. A sleep schedule based on that old maxim, however, will improve your resistance to stress.

▸ Have sex. Sex is an excellent antidote for stress. (Unless what you have to go through to have sex is itself prohibitively stressful.)

Wherever and Whenever

▸ Limit your intake of alcohol and caffeine. Your body's reaction to the chemicals in those substances doesn't lower your stress levels, it raises them.

▸ Go with the flow. You know there are unavoidable situations and conditions, and people who annoy, anger, or frustrate you. Accept your fate. Shrug your shoulders, relax, and let those stressful emotions drift away. (You don't have to grin, but you do have to bear it.)

▶ Exercise regularly. Brisk physical activity is one of the best stress reme-
dies available. In addition to forcing you to take time for yourself, exercise relaxes you, increases alertness, clears your mind, allows you to
sleep longer and deeper, renews energy, removes toxins, and improves
circulation. And the endorphins released during exercise elevate your
spirits and dramatically improve your health. Stretching exercises are
also fine stress relievers. Try slowly stretching your neck, shoulders, and
legs the next time you feel stress, pressure, or anxiety creeping up on you.

Case Histories

When Chicago Bears running back Walter Payton died, dozens of elite
athletes shared memories of their fallen hero. Although the late Hall of
Famer's career was rich in unprecedented achievements and incredible
records, it quickly became evident that what most inspired the men who
knew him was Payton's unmatched dedication to his craft. Every off season for more than a decade, Walter Payton conditioned himself by sprinting up and down a steep jagged hill near his home. Despite his family
obligations and his hands-on involvement in several businesses and char-
ities, Payton found the time to hit that vicious hill hard every day. He
wanted to become the best running back ever, and through sheer effort as
much as natural talent, he did.

Walter Payton's amazing work ethic inspired hundreds of young gridiron
warriors, and rightly so. Who, I wondered, would best inspire "civilians"
like you? Who can average, everyday people trying to become fit and
healthy use as a role model?

How about other average, everyday people who made commitments and
sustained efforts, and reached their goals?

Maria

Maria was a beautiful baby who grew into a lively, funny, intelligent child.
Until she became a teenager, Maria was lean and athletic. By the time she
reached her junior year in high school, however, Maria was obese, weigh-
ing nearly 200 pounds. And she was frequently ill, constantly beset with
colds, uncontrollable allergies, and chronic fatigue. A constant target of

teasing and scorn from classmates, Maria developed deep-seated feelings of inferiority and depression.

One day Maria looked at herself in the mirror and decided she'd simply had enough embarrassment, abuse, and fat jokes to last her the rest of her life. I helped her design a fat reduction plan very similar to the one I'm recommending to you. Within one year Maria lost sixty-two pounds. Her dress size dropped from 18 to 6. I'm sure my advice helped Maria, but let's be clear: She did it herself—despite her academic obligations and despite living with an overweight, unhealthy single mom who was unable to offer much support. Maria is beautiful again, and all the charm, wit, and humor so evident in her childhood has returned. Her range of activities has expanded dramatically, and lately she's been indulging her interest in karate.

Brian

An extremely successful businessman, Brian played golf several days each week. Golf made Brian thirsty, so he drank as he golfed. Beer out on the course, martinis or scotch in the clubhouse, more when he got home.

When Brian got married at age twenty-eight, he weighed 170 pounds. As his business grew, so did his body. Ten years later Brian weighed over 200—a sloppy, badly distributed burden. Thick jowls hung from his bloated face, and his waistline resembled a radial tire melting in the sun.

When two of his college friends dropped dead in their late thirties and early forties, Brian decided it was time to make some serious changes in his lifestyle. After six months on my fat reduction program, Brain looked like a college quarterback. His doctor was so impressed with Brian's new body that he wondered if Brian was using steroids. Brian's lean muscle mass and metabolic rate have increased dramatically, and his LDL and blood sugar levels are way down. His improved strength allows Brian to drive a golf ball fifty yards farther then he ever did before, and he has no trouble keeping up with his three very active daughters. Simply by dedicating himself to change, Brian has remodeled his body and his entire life. He still plays golf frequently, but now his beverages of choice are mineral water and fruit juice.

Caroline

An ex-smoker and a recovering alcoholic, Caroline recently had a baby. Determined to rid herself of the seventy pounds she had put on during her pregnancy, Caroline went on a low-calorie diet and signed up for aerobics classes. But Caroline is a working mom. The pace and pressure imposed by her dual role soon forced her to give up the aerobics classes, and the low-calorie diet wasn't really working out.

By the time her baby was eight months old, Caroline was, in her own words, "a complete mess." After studying my fat reduction advice, Caroline concluded that she might be able to put together a nutrition and exercise plan that would fit into her busy life.

She was right. In less than a year Caroline lost forty-five pounds of excess fat. She calls my No-Excuses Workout "a great way to set up the whole day." Caroline describes her early morning NEW as "my daily refresher and body makeover."

Sam

A classroom full of hyperactive preteens is probably not the best place for a stressed-out, overweight fifty-four-year-old to spend his days, but that's where Sam finds himself, Monday through Friday, ten months a year. "These kids are driving me nuts," Sam told me. "I'm completely wiped out at the end of the day."

I suggested that Sam give my fat reduction system a try, and after enduring a little nagging, he did. Now, four months later, Sam's waistline has shrunk three inches. More important, he shows up for work rested, refreshed, and full of energy. Although he hasn't been tested recently, I'll bet Sam's stress levels have declined significantly. He's certainly nowhere near as frazzled and edgy as he used to be.

Rebecca

When Rebecca returned home from the hospital after an emergency appendectomy, Dwight, the man she'd been living with for more than three years, was gone. So was the television, the VCR, the microwave, and some furniture. "I felt as if my life had turned into a bad country song," Rebecca told me.

Devastated, Rebecca turned to food for comfort. Lots of food. The richest, nastiest, greasiest food she could get. Already a shade too wide and a tad too round, Rebecca soon found herself carrying around an additional sixty pounds.

A chance meeting with a friend she hadn't seen in years woke Rebecca up. "At first Linda didn't even recognize me," Rebecca recalls. "Then as we talked, I could see how uncomfortable I was making her. The pity or disgust or whatever it was I saw in her eyes convinced me it was time to quit feeling sorry for myself and get my big ass in gear."

Rebecca's crusade to rid herself of excess fat began with three months of devotion to my fat-burning system. Then she branched out to step aerobics. Today she works out three or four times a week. Whenever the opportunity presents itself, she skates or plays beach volleyball. And she eats whatever she wants—which isn't nearly as much as she once thought she needed to survive the post-Dwight era.

Emily

Last year Emily, eighty-two at the time, had open heart surgery. If she wanted to stay alive, Emily's doctors told her, she was going to have to exercise to strengthen her heart. I designed a gentle low-impact version of the NEW that Emily has followed carefully and conscientiously for several months now.

I heard from Emily about a week ago. She is thrilled about how sharp and lively she feels and is "amazed" at how much better she looks. Most important, according to Emily, she has fun with her grandkids again.

The thousands of men and women who have recharged, streamlined, and reshaped their bodies using the same strategies you'll be applying soon come from all over the country, from all walks of life, and from a wide range of professions, lifestyles, and backgrounds. Our roster of successful fat burners includes thousands of people like Maria, Brian, Caroline, Sam, Rebecca, and Emily. Some found it relatively easy to blend their fat reduction efforts into their daily lives; others found it much tougher. Some attacked their challenge with relish and enthusiasm, others with reluctance or grim determination. Some crushed the obstacles that life placed before them, while others struggled to stay on course.

But they all reached their goals. They were strong and smart when they needed to be, and now they're gliding along in lean new bodies they built themselves.

You can, too.

C H A P T E R 6

The 30-Day
Meltdown

Professional sports teams rely on lengthy, carefully structured training camps to prepare their athletes for the rigors and demands of formal competition. Tightly focused practice sessions and conditioning drills hone techniques and strengthen bodies. Hours of meetings and one-on-one discussions deepen understanding and build motivation. Long nights of study and analysis sharpen minds.

The value of this extended preseason training is obvious, and the necessity for it unquestioned. Without adequate preparation it's impossible for the athletes to perform anywhere near peak levels. Not even the most talented competitor can shrug off weeks or months of inactivity and indulgence overnight. No matter how gifted he is, no NBA point guard can step off the golf course and onto a basketball court and be ready to play an eighty-two-game season. No matter how clever or how quick she is, no world-class volleyball player can go directly from sunning by the beach to the volleyball court and expect to survive the first half of her team's first game.

To ensure a successful launch of your fat-burning crusade, you, too, need a training camp—a transitional period during which you condition your body and your mind to understand and accept the new eating and exercise habits you are striving to establish.

Few human beings like change, and we really hate harsh, abrupt disruption of familiar routines. Gradual one-step-at-a-time implementation of new behaviors is a much more effective and far easier way to go—which is why your kick-start countdown lasts thirty days, not thirty minutes.

Do a little something each day, and each day will bring you closer to maximum fat-burning efficiency and the body you want.

Day 1: Systems Check I

Complete the self-assessment tests in Chapter 2. Record your scores. Regardless of how you fare in the tests, don't be depressed, discouraged, or angry. Place no judgment on yourself. The tests are simply an objective measure of your starting line, not an indictment of your character or lifestyle. Don't waste your time and energy berating yourself for whatever you think you did over the months or years to weaken or soften or thicken your body.

Placing blame is a loser's game. Instead of becoming entangled and immobilized by the why's and how's of your problem, adopt a solution-oriented approach to fat loss. You will stop looking back to your past. Who cares where your excess fat came from, because it will soon be gone? Look to the future, where you'll be spending the rest of your life.

If you like, start a journal to keep track of your progress. And have a "before" photo taken or record a video of yourself. If it pleases you to know that your body will look and feel a little better every day from now on, smile and say: "Lean!"

Day 2: A Wake-up Call

Get your body out of bed a few minutes earlier than you usually do. March in place (NEW exercise #1) for two or three minutes. Don't apply the force or exertion the instructions call for just yet. Maintain an easy, relaxed rhythm. When you're warm and loose, complete one flexibility routine circuit (see pages 79–83) slowly. Use a languid pace and pay attention to your form and breathing. Don't strain or rock into position. Slowly stretch as far out, up, or down as you can. Hold your full extension for several seconds.

An hour or so before dinner, practice your seven-minute routine. Do each exercise once or twice, or until you're familiar with each movement and comfortable with your mechanics. Go slowly and take as much time as you need to become comfortable with each exercise. Pay close attention to form and balance. If something you do causes sudden pain or discomfort, or if some specific movement just doesn't feel right, reread the instructions and study the photos.

Don't exert yourself in either the stretching or NEW orientation. (You're not working out yet.)

Day 3: Wash Away Your Toxins

Resolve to drink at least 64 ounces of bottled water every day. Tap or fountain water is acceptable, but only when spring water or filtered water is not convenient. If you're currently wasting your money on sugary soda and artificial juices, buy spring water by the case instead. (Those giant wholesale food depots will sell you a garageful of the stuff for pennies a bottle.)

Carry a water bottle with you wherever you go. Sip from it frequently even if you don't feel particularly thirsty. Drinking water only when you're thirsty is like waiting for your gas tank to empty completely before you fill it.

Water removes metabolic wastes and other toxins from the body, minimizes hunger, and aids the fat-burning process significantly. Despite what you may have read or heard, you can—and should—drink water with your meals.

For your morning exercise today, warm up with a couple of minutes of marching in place. Stretch gently. Try to do ten push-ups followed by ten crunches. If you can't handle ten repetitions of each exercise without strain, do as many as you can. Before dinner, take a walk—not a fitness walk or a power walk, just a walk. Stroll easily to start. When you feel loose and warm, pick up the pace just a bit. Don't exert yourself but simply walk briskly for about ten minutes.

Day 4: Visualization

Daydream a little. Find a quiet corner and use your mind to fast-forward a few months. See and feel your new body and experience what you're going to do with it. See yourself wading in a South Pacific lagoon or navigating the rambling canyon passes of Utah. See yourself gliding around the dance floor or fitting comfortably into an airplane seat.

Use guided imagery to launch powerful mental assaults on particularly annoying fat clusters. Numerous studies published in medical journals have validated the success of cancer patients who used similar search-and-destroy imagery to shrink or eradicate malignant tumors.

If you think your imaging efforts might work better with external stimuli, flip through magazines and catalogs to find pictures of the kind of body you'd like to be walking around in. (And while you're browsing, take note of all the great clothes you'll be able to wear comfortably and confidently in a few weeks.)

For your morning exercise, complete your first No-Excuses Workout. One circuit only. Move briskly and steadily, but don't go full throttle just yet. Half or three-quarter speed is sufficient to introduce your body to this new level of activity.

Day 5: Planning

Some people are meticulous planners. They script every element of every project they take on. Others concentrate on their goals with a more instinctual, less regimented attitude. Each camp would do well to appreciate and adopt useful aspects of the other's outlook.

You analytical task-oriented folks should certainly plan every phase of your fat reduction effort in any level of detail you like. Create menus for each meal and snack using the charts on pages 45–47. Schedule exercise by time, location, and type of activity. That's fine. But, hey, things happen. So be flexible. If real life intrudes upon your master plan (and it will), don't panic. There are hundreds of acceptable substitutes for the foods you plan to eat next Tuesday at 6:08 P.M. And there are lots of seven-, fourteen-, and twenty-eight-minute blocks of time available when you need to reschedule your NEW exercise sessions. Keep your mind on your goal; don't be overly concerned about the precise path you'll take to get there.

You "seat of the pants, let's see what the day brings" types are going to have to recognize and acknowledge the need for important eating and exercise parameters. Until healthy nutrition and activity behaviors become unconscious habit, you need some kind of a plan. So make one. Schedule exercise and come up with at least a general idea of what you'll be eating over the next few days.

No NEW today. If you like, a short warm-up and some stretching would be nice, or maybe a casual walk before or after dinner.

Day 6: Fat-Burning Meals

To burn fat quickly during this kick-start period, your meals should consist almost entirely of lean proteins and fibrous carbs (see Chapter 3). For example, have a low-fat cheese and herb omelet with tomatoes for breakfast, but skip the toast and hash browns. For lunch, take your cheeseburger off its bun and eat it with a mixed green salad instead of curly fries.

This is an NEW day—one circuit in the morning before breakfast. Push yourself just a little this time by revving up the intensity for two or three of the exercises.

Day 7: Your Window of Opportunity

Remain simple-carb-vigilant during the day, but for your evening Window of Opportunity Meal (W/O Meal), eat anything you want. Use your trusty dinner plate to keep portion size within reason and to maintain nutritional balance. Remember to start your meal with a colorful crunchy salad. Consume equal portions of lean protein (meat, fish, poultry), fibrous carbs (veggies), and simple carbs (cake, pie, wine, flavored yogurt). If you want seconds, take a little of everything, in equal proportion. Whatever you decide to eat, be sure that your W/O Meal lasts no longer than one hour from start to finish.

No NEW today, but stretching and walking are certainly encouraged.

Day 8: Take Your Body to the Movies

Rent some inspirational videos of the "hopeless underdog somehow emerges victorious" genre. Try *Rocky* (the original), *Breaking Away, Rudy, Enough,* or *Hoosiers* (apparently a lot of inspiring activity goes on almost nonstop in the state of Indiana) or any other movie you know of that chronicles an average man or woman's heartbreaking struggle against—and ultimate triumph over—seemingly insurmountable obstacles.

Band of Brothers, a ten-part series produced by the cable channel HBO, is a serious and profoundly humbling study of a group of everyday American farmers, postal workers, factory workers, and clerks who conquered hunger, exhaustion, and the constant possibility of imminent death to end Hitler's oppression of Europe. If this true World War II story doesn't offer some role models you can connect with, no movie will.

As you watch the ordinary people who are the heroes of these films scratch and fight toward their goals, make an effort to truly appreciate their efforts and resolve to emulate the focus, will, and spirit that drives them onward.

It's another NEW day. You're starting to look forward to putting your body through its paces, aren't you?

Day 9: What's Cooking?

Get into that kitchen and rattle those pots and pans. Prepare a meal from entirely fresh ingredients. Look through Chapter 8 or survey your own recipe files for dishes that excite your curiosity or tweak your taste buds. Serve your meal as if it came from the kitchen of a fine restaurant.

Consume your masterpiece slowly and gratefully. Appreciate and savor all its textures, aromas, and nuances.

Food is good, isn't it?

And good food is even better.

No NEW today, but if you're feeling restless, your walking shoes await, or do some stretching exercises.

Day 10: Churn and Burn

By now your body's starting to like your NEW. Maybe it wants a little more. In your morning session today, add a burst of effort and explosion to every other exercise. Remind yourself that varying intensity levels in your workouts keeps your metabolism from slipping into its cruise control mode.

You'll never have total control over your metabolism; no one does. Age and genetics will always play some role in determining how much fat you can burn and how quickly you can burn it. You can, however, use my Variable Intensity Training (VIT) principles to increase your metabolic rate dramatically.

Day 11: Give Teas a Chance

Green tea is rich in antioxidants—those powerful disease-prevention substances that help your body rid itself of dangerous toxins. Black tea, recent studies indicate, boosts metabolic rates slightly (to the tune of about 80 calories a day).

Both teas are excellent alternatives to the sugar-and-fat-laced designer coffees now available on every street corner in every city, town, village, and hamlet in the nation.

So try some tea, hot or iced, straight up or with a lemon wedge and a squirt of honey. You might like it.

No NEW today, but if your body wants some gentle stretching and walking around, go for it.

Day 12: Snack Smart

If hunger strikes between meals or if you simply feel and function better when you reduce meal portions to allow for preplanned snacks throughout the day, remember to limit your intake of sugary, fat-tainted simple carbs. A handful of almonds, walnuts, or cashews (lightly salted or unsalted, of course) won't hurt your fat reduction efforts a bit. In fact, the monounsaturated oils in these nuts are actually good for you.

Chapter 8 offers a variety of tasty and satisfying low-carb snacks you can enjoy confidently. (Try the Turkey Wraps on page 169.) And you should always feel free to consume all the raw veggies you can get your hands on.

Today's an NEW day. One in the morning, before breakfast. If you feel ambitious, add one circuit before dinner. Fourteen minutes of resuscitation and stress relief—and it's completely legal. Don't forget to vary the intensity of every other exercise.

Day 13: Relax

Is your inbox overflowing? Will printing your e-mail take an hour and a half? Is your boss following you around the job site like a rabid angry stalker? Is your mate on your case? Are your kids on your nerves? Is your neck stiff, your back tight, your stomach in knots?

Sounds like some stress reduction exercises are in order. Find a quiet corner and practice one or both of the following stress-fighting techniques:

Deep breathing involves filling and emptying your upper and lower lungs through waves of deep breathing. Inhale slowly and deeply through your nose. Hold for two or three seconds. Exhale completely through your mouth. Refill your lungs. Empty slowly and completely. Repeat, rolling one breath into the next. In. Out. As you exhale, feel the tension leaving your body.

Progressive muscle relaxation is a process you can use to train all your muscles to relax at once. A three-part technique is used. Starting with your toes and slowly working your way up, isolate, tense, and relax first small muscle groups, then larger groups, and, finally, entire areas. Your body will learn to accept and act upon your relaxation signal after only a couple of sessions.

No NEW today, but maybe you'll come across a bike that needs riding.

Day 14: Boost Your Nutrition

Explore the wide wonderful world of nutritional supplements. Begin with the brief sketches offered in Chapter 3. If you find a substance that you think might be useful in your fat-burning efforts, investigate its pedigree. Go online or talk to those eager friendly folks at the health food store.

If you do use a supplement, remember that the best time to take most nutritional aids is with meals. Absorption will occur more quickly and thoroughly, giving your tissues access to the supplement's benefits in a timely, natural fashion.

Today's an NEW day. VIT in the morning and VIT at night makes all of us fat burners lean, strong, and tight. (An irresistible compulsion to rhyme came over me.)

Day 15: Turn Up the Music

The clever people who run Las Vegas casinos discovered years ago that music has a significant effect on activity and energy levels. Lively happy tunes are piped into gambling venues all day and all night to keep customers alert and playing—and playing noticeably faster than they do *sans* tunes. The math of the casino biz being pretty much immutable, the faster players play, the more money the casino earns.

Even if you don't own a casino (or a pinkie ring), you, too, can profit from music's direct effect on movement and attitude. Create an exercise soundtrack built around a strong beat and pleasant rhythms. If you can't find a radio station that meets your needs and nothing in your CD collection is quite right, either, put together your own workout mixes. The library offers a great selection.

Start your tape or CD with gentle medium-beat tunes (for warm-up and stretching), then change to firm upbeat selections for the heart of your workout. Bring the beat down to cool off. You can also vary the tempo in your mix's central section to mimic VIT principles. Alternate medium-fast pop or country with full-tilt rock or salsa, and you'll find that you have created "variable intensity music."

It's fun to make your own mixes, but if you'd rather avoid the hassle, there are plenty of premixed workout tapes and CDs available.

No NEW today. Got any leaves to rake, grass to cut, snow to shovel? How about the dog? Does Spot need a run?

Day 16: Boost Your Nutrition

The U.S. Department of Health and Human Services insists that unhealthy eating habits cause more cancer deaths each year than smoking. While the average American's diet does tend to be too high in fat and salt, and too low in fiber, our primary dietary problem, health experts point out, is a severe deficiency of the phyto-nutrients obtained from fruits and vegetables.

Resolve to consume more fruits and vegetables each and every day. These foods are generally high in fiber, low in fat, and rich in vitamins, minerals, enzymes and antioxidants. For example, make a serious effort to snack on crisp raw carrots and celery instead of cookies and chips.

Chapter 8 is stocked with dozens of suggestions for fitting fruits and vegetables into your daily eating plan. You'll find an array of entrées, soups, salads, side dishes, and snacks. Use these recipes or create your own. One way or another, bring more fruits and vegetables into your life. Your body really needs the nutrients they provide.

It's a NEW day with VIT, early and late.

Day 17: The Low-Cost, High-Value Mini-Workout

Exercise scientists recently discovered that men and women who exercised even for a few minutes two or three times a week enjoyed most of the health and fitness benefits normally obtained from a traditional workout program. If my math is correct, that's a four-to-one improvement on the effort invested.

You can add value to your exercise program simply by adding a few minutes of well-paced movement and activity to your everyday schedule.

For example, if you drive to work, park in the most remote corner of the employee lot. Walk briskly to the front door. If you use public transportation to get to your job, get off a stop early and walk the rest of the way. Or walk around the block for a few minutes before you go in. Always prefer stairways to elevators or escalators. Dismiss your lawn service and do the work yourself. Ride your bike to the bank or the video store. Walk to church, the movies, and the library.

You get the idea. Examine your daily routine. Find ways to fit in some vigorous physical activity beyond your formal workouts. You'll reach your fat reduction goals much more quickly.

No NEW today, but maybe what you just read will spark some extra-credit exercise initiative.

Day 18: Eat Peanut Butter

The fats and oils in peanut butter aid muscle growth, boost good cholesterol levels, and strengthen the heart. The next time a snack attack strikes, spread some peanut or almond butter on celery stalks, apple wedges, or a cracker.

Today's a NEW day. Push it early, push it late. You're getting stronger and leaner; you know you are.

Day 19: Get a Massage

Treat yourself to a therapeutic massage. A professional massage therapist will offer numerous techniques including Deep Tissue, Shiatsu, or Swedish, just to name a few. The magic emanating from trained hands will improve your circulation, reduce your stress levels, aid in the repair and regeneration of muscle tissue, and promote efficient waste disposal. Drink lots of water afterward to flush the impurities from your body.

If you can't afford a professional massage, maybe your mate can be convinced that you've earned a little pampering.

No NEW today. Relax. Okay, stretch if you want to.

Day 20: Be Prepared

Hey, you're ten days from the conclusion of your kick-start training camp. This is a good time to start looking ahead. Think about the immediate future. Do you see any obvious obstacles standing between you and your fitness goals? Is there a vacation or a holiday or a big family function coming up? Any other potential occasions of sin on the horizon? Will the weather soon become a factor in your supplemental exercise plans? Is there someone close to you who seems to resent your commitment to change? Identify potential pitfalls and devise effective countermeasures. Keep your hands on the wheel and your feet on the floor. Stay on course.

It's a NEW day, the last before your first evaluation milestone. Give it your best shot.

Day 21: Systems Check II

Retake the self-assessment tests described in Chapter 2. Compare your results to those you recorded after your initial systems check. Congratulate yourself if you see any improvement in your scores. However, if your scores are not as good as you hoped, review your eating and exercise behaviors. Decide what needs fixing and resolve to fix it. If you determine that your behaviors have been pretty much on target, relax. Keep doing what you've been doing. Everyone's metabolism is unique. Even if your scores don't yet reflect it, I assure you that something good is happening deep inside your body's cellular structures.

No NEW today. I'll leave you to your own devices. If one of those devices happens to be a stationary bike or a jump rope, you know what to do.

Day 22: Why Weights?

Strength-building exercise has the power to keep your metabolism active around the clock. Weight and resistance training can turn weak, flaccid muscles into powerful fat-burning incinerators.

If you don't constantly build up your muscles, the aging process will shrink them. Each pound of muscle mass you lose through neglect or inactivity reduces your body's fat-burning capacity by 35 to 50 calories a day.

Fortunately, you can use weight or resistance exercises to build and maintain your valuable muscle mass. The NEW is already designed to include the benefits of resistance training. However, you might want to experiment with some light dumbbells or wear ankle weights during your NEW circuit. Excellent books and Web sites are available to help you lift safely and effectively. (See the Resource Guide on pages 177–181.)

It's a NEW day. How many reps can you do for each exercise?

Day 23: Go Shopping

Create a complete menu for the next seven to ten days. Use the recipes in Chapter 8 and your own favorites as sources. Then go shopping for the supplies you'll need to prepare those meals. Try to fill your grocery cart with lean protein, fresh fruit, vegetables, spices, and herbs. Be adventurous.

No NEW today. Go for a brisk walk if you insist.

Day 24: Get a Hobby

Several studies have shown conclusively that hobbies are much more than pleasant diversions. Hobbies, it turns out, have a calming, restorative effect on our bodies and minds, lowering blood pressure and increasing our levels of seratonin—a neurotransmitter associated with feelings of well-being.

So what do you like to do in your free time? Photography? Sewing? Woodworking? Gardening? Painting? Whatever it is, make time to do it; your stress levels will plummet.

It's a NEW day. You are now burning fat night and day.

Day 25: More C Anyone?

Researchers at the National Institutes of Health say that our daily intake of vitamin C should be doubled or tripled. Why? Because C's health benefits are impressive. This nutrient stimulates antibodies that fight infection, helps stop the production of cancer-causing nitrosamines in the stomach, assists in ridding the body of stored toxins, and improves our ability to absorb and use calcium. Most important, there is evidence that the antioxidants in vitamin C prevent the free radical damage that often leads to cancer and tumor growth.

You probably already know that citrus fruits (oranges, grapefruit, tangerines) and tomatoes are rich in C. You may not realize that fruits such as cantaloupe, honeydew melon, kiwi, mango, papaya, pineapple, raspberries, strawberries, and watermelon are excellent sources as well. And let's not forget about vegetables such as asparagus, broccoli, Brussels sprouts, cabbage, cauliflower, kale, mustard greens, peppers, snow peas, and sweet potatoes.

No NEW today. How's that jogging thing going? Or was it a stationary bike spin?

Day 26: Find a Partner

See if you can interest your spouse or a friend in joining your exercise program. Put together a mutually convenient workout schedule and burn some fat together. You're less likely to become lazy or indifferent when you know someone else is counting on you for encouragement, motivation, and support. If your spouse becomes your partner, plan, prepare, and eat your meals together. What a great bonding experience.

It's a NEW day. Two circuits, please, A.M. and P.M.

Day 27: Expand Your Exercise Arsenal

Your body is an efficiency expert. Repeat the same exercise routine at the same pace day after day, and your body will soon learn how to burn less and less energy to complete its work.

To continue progressing rapidly toward your fat reduction goals, you're going to have to shake up your workout regimen every six weeks or so. Change the order of your exercises, work out longer or harder. Every week or two, substitute any aerobic activity for one NEW circuit. Remember to use a VIT strategy. Chapter 7 is full of suggestions to help you expand and diversify your activity options.

No NEW today, but experiment with some exercise alternatives.

Day 28: Be Curious, Alert, Interested

Surf the net or browse health and fitness periodicals to keep yourself up to date on all the latest fat-burning news. Read those pamphlets the local hospital or your insurance company is always sending. Collect and save healthy recipes, workout tips, and research results you can use. The Resource Guide on pages 177–181 will steer you in the right direction.

It's a NEW day. Getting routine, isn't it?

Day 29: Systems Check III

As you ready yourself for the transition from kick-start to steady lifelong burn, complete the self-assessment tests in Chapter 2 one more time. Compare today's scores to your initial numbers and to your intermediate scores as well. You should see clear evidence of a positive trend. If you don't, review your exercise and eating behaviors critically and objectively. If you discover flaws in your strategy or lapses in execution, resolve to correct those flaws. Throw back your shoulders and move on. If you can't locate the causes of your disappointing performance immediately, check out the troubleshooting section in Chapter 7.

No NEW today. Do you feel like pumping some hand weights or pedaling an exercise bike while you watch TV?

Day 30: Ignition

Congratulations! You've made it through training camp. You are now a full-fledged, officially certified fat burner. No diploma or decoder ring commemorates your accomplishment; you'll have to settle for the pride, satisfaction, and self-respect you've earned through sheer effort and commitment.

Celebrate the end of your kick-start phase with a little victory dance of your own design (clothing and other participants optional). Go on to Chapter 7 for suggestions and recommendations that may help you improve and enlarge upon what you've learned.

It's a NEW day. You know what to do. And now that you're clearly in charge, it's time to revisit the NEW frequency schedule discussed in detail in Chapter 4. Push yourself up the intensity ladder you'll find on page 127 whenever you feel yourself becoming too comfortable with your routine. Stay focused. You've come too far to backslide now.

7

A Fitness
Operator's Manual

The phone rang.

It was Dave, a real estate broker I met through a friend of a friend. About six weeks prior to his call, Dave had decided to give my fat-burning system what he called "an honest shot." After a couple of false starts, Dave got it all together. He ate wisely and followed my exercise recommendations carefully and consistently. Now he was nearing the end of his thirty-day kick-start effort.

"I have a progress report for you," Dave told me. "I'm down fourteen pounds. Feeling good. Looking good. The beer belly's almost gone, and I think I see what might be muscle all through my arms and upper body."

"Congratulations," I said.

"Yeah, thanks," said Dave. "So what now?"

An excellent question. And judging from the feedback I've gotten over the years, this question has an apparently unlimited supply of answers.

About 10 to 15 percent of my fat-burning "graduates" use their thirty-day kick-start as a springboard to an intense regimen of physical activity (mountain climbing, cross-country skiing, long-distance hiking) or serious amateur athletics (rugby, soccer, hockey, organized basketball).

Another 30 percent or so find that the eating and exercise plans they developed as they worked through the fat-burning process provide everything they need to maintain a satisfactory level of health and fitness. Their answer to Dave's "what now" question frequently is: "More of the same. I don't cringe anymore when I pass a mirror, I can keep up with the kids in the park or on vacation, and my mate doesn't shudder when I get a certain gleam in my eye. I'm doing just fine, thank you very much."

About half of the men and women who complete my thirty-day program eventually add some sort of regular exercise to their daily lives in addition to or in place of our No-Excuses Workout. Why? Because they discover that they want to. They enjoy their new bodies and take every opportunity to use them.

If you trade in your four-year-old minivan for a new Porsche, your attitude about driving would probably change radically. Replace your soft, slow body with a sleeker, trimmer frame, and a similar outlook adjustment is likely to occur.

The International Sports Sciences Association recommends at least twenty minutes of exercise at least three times a week to maintain acceptable fitness levels. My No-Excuses Workout is an effective and convenient method of meeting that requirement, but like a new car buyer intrigued with all the high-performance options described so seductively in those slick color brochures, a considerable number of our fat burners see some upgrades they want and decide that they're willing to pay a little extra to get them. They go beyond my NEW not only because a variety of physical activities is good for them, but because it feels good and offers new challenges. They exercise to clear their heads or reduce their stress levels, or for additional strength or endurance or muscle definition—or for the pure joy of it.

Expanding Your Horizons

Depending upon what you want to use your new body for, your age and physical capabilities, the time you have available, and the amount of money you're willing to spend, there are several viable exercise options you might soon find yourself seriously considering. Some are conditioning or toning regimens, others are recreational activities.

Physical fitness is a personal process. The Resource Guide on pages 177–181 will help you find your way to all the information you need to design and direct your own unique exercise program. You may find that fitness walking is an excellent complement to my No-Excuses Workout, especially if you incorporate Variable Intensity Training principles. A few weeks of walking may lead to jogging or running. Maybe step aerobics will appeal to you, or cardio-boxing or swimming or schoolyard basketball or weight training or mountain biking or roller-skating. The possibilities are limited only by your schedule, your sense of adventure, and your budget.

I can offer some guidelines that you may find useful if and when you decide to explore the wide range of exercise options widely available.

▶ Start your exercise program (whatever it may be) at your own pace. Increase your program gradually. You'll probably feel the urge to get going full throttle as quickly as possible. Please control that impulse. There is an adaptation sequence that must play itself out before the body completely adjusts to new patterns of activity. Once an adequate conditioning period has passed, you can seek tougher challenges. If you've been fitness walking three days a week for a month and decide you'd like to include some jogging in each of your outings, follow a phase-in routine something like this:

> Week 1: Fifteen minutes walking; five minutes jogging
> Week 2: Ten minutes walking; ten minutes jogging
> Week 3: Five minutes walking; fifteen minutes jogging
> Week 4: Five minutes walking; fifteen minutes jogging

▶ Always warm up before exercising and cool down afterward. A short walk, light jog, marching in place, or a few minutes on a stationary bike followed by gentle stretching of your legs, back, shoulders, and trunk loosens your muscles and lubricates your joints.

▶ If you're in some sort of group activity, don't feel obligated to perform at the pace of others. Compete only with yourself. Strive to be just a little better with each workout.

▶ Accept the fact that on some days you simply won't be able to perform as well as you'd like. Not even a premier athlete's body is equally willing every day. Pay attention when your body rebels, but come back fresh and eager for your next session.

▶ If you don't look forward to your exercise sessions, try some other activity option. Find a routine or sport you enjoy. There's no law against exercise being fun.

▶ Include as many different activities as you can in your overall exercise plan. Mixing and matching a number of aerobic and anaerobic workouts will enhance the value of each.

▶ If something you're doing hurts, stop. Listen to your body.

▶ Be consistent in your scheduling. A workout every two or three weeks is not only useless, it could be dangerous. Sudden exertion can tear up an unprepared body.

▶ Turbocharge your aerobic activities with high-energy "bursts." The Variable Intensity Training approach will add substantial calorie-burning benefits to any aerobic workout.

▶ Don't allow yourself to become dehydrated during exercise. Drink water (the fluid your body absorbs best) before, during, and after each workout.

The Fitness Mega Mall

Let's imagine it's three or four months from now. Your antifat nutritional strategy has evolved into a firmly fixed habit. You've mastered my No-Excuses Workout and all its variations. You look great and feel terrific. And yet you're not quite satisfied. You feel the need for a wider variety of activities and maybe some tougher challenges to sustain your interest and enthusiasm.

So you page through the Resource Guide, visit the library, talk with your active friends, and surf the net. Before you can learn to spell kinesiology, you find yourself facing an overwhelming array of activity choices.

How do you sort through the blizzard of "expert" advice, infomercial hyperbole, and evangelical program recommendations that will bury you the moment you exhibit an interest in any aspect of physical fitness? How will you find a fitness approach compatible with your preferences, goals, schedule, and budget?

"Join a health club," says my friend Joe.

Because Joe manages an excellent health and fitness center in a Chicago suburb, he is, of course, not an entirely objective source of advice. He does, however, raise some valid issues.

"If you want a choice of the latest movies, you go to one of those thirty-screen Cineplexes," Joe says. "If you want to get your Christmas shopping done without driving all over three counties, you head for the closest mega mall. And if you want a smart, convenient way to get regular access to a wide range of workout options and fitness machinery, you really should investigate a health club membership."

A well-run health club, Joe contends, offers something for everyone. "If you like power walking or jogging, you'll like it more on a shock absorbent composition track or treadmill where it's pretty unlikely you'll get struck by lightning or bitten by a Doberman or hit by a truck," he says. "And unless you're wealthy, there's no way you can afford—or have space for—all the different kinds of strength and aerobic equipment you'll find at a decent health club. Where else can you go to jog on Monday, hit the weight circuit on Tuesday, take a low-impact aerobics class on Wednesday, cross-country ski on Thursday, and play racquetball on Saturday? And where else will you find people who can show you how to do all those things without hurting yourself?"

If Joe's thinly disguised sales pitch makes sense to you, a health club membership may indeed be an idea worth exploring at some time. Before you sign on any dotted lines, though, remember that health club dues can run from a few hundred to well over a thousand dollars annually. Approach the purchase of a membership the same way you would any other invest-ment. Analyze the cost/benefit ratio in relation to your goals and needs.

Here are some factors to consider:

▶ Not all health clubs are alike, so shop around. Some clubs emphasize strength training, while others offer a wider choice of aerobic or circuit training. Choose a club compatible with your interests and fitness goals.

▶ Be comfortable. A young woman may not enjoy a club full of big, crusty bodybuilders, and a middle-aged man may feel out of place in a club overrun with young, rowdy hard bodies.

▶ Require professionalism. The club should be clean, well cared for, and run by upbeat accessible personnel. An adequate supply of up-to-date and well-maintained equipment should be on hand. Trainers should be certified by a nationally recognized organization and be able to help you with all aspects of fitness: strength, cardiovascular maintenance, and flexibility. If a club purports to offer training in a special-interest activity such as boxing or racquetball, staffers should be competent instructors in those fields as well.

▶ Try before you buy. Request a guest pass and work out a couple of times before making any financial commitment.

▶ Evaluate atmosphere and amenities. Do you require the luxury and frills of a big-time club, or will you be more comfortable in a basic gym/track setting? If massages, a pool, and a steam room are important to you, make sure they're important to your club, too.

▶ Find a club near home or work or halfway in between. If you have to go too far out of your way to get to the club, you'll soon tire of the inconvenience.

▶ Keep the length of your contract as short as possible and negotiate reasonable termination options.

If you find a club that meets your standards and addresses your needs, remember that it's up to you to get your money's worth. Keep up with club offerings, which often change over time. Read the bulletin boards to learn about classes or outings that may interest you. These announcement boards are also sometimes excellent sources for nutrition and exercise tips and, from time to time, equipment deals. (Be skeptical about nutritional supplements offered for sale at the club. You can usually find better prices for similar items in retail outlets, by mail order, or on the Internet.

Above all, visit your club regularly and take full advantage of the variety of activities available. Remember that easy access to a wide spectrum of workout choices is the main reason you joined the club in the first place. And use the trainers you're paying for to ensure that you are exercising properly and safely.

Troubleshooting

All new car models ever introduced, all plant renovation projects ever undertaken, and all new computers ever built have something in common—several things, in fact: setbacks, glitches, missteps, and delays. Unless you're blessed with extraordinary concentration and self-control, you shouldn't be surprised if you encounter a problem or two as your fat reduction effort unfolds.

You'll be well on your way to the new body you're striving to build, eating wisely and exercising regularly. Then one day you'll lose focus. You'll become overconfident, distracted by some special event, or waylaid by some traumatic occurrence. For whatever reason, you'll stray from the path of righteousness and return briefly to the evil kingdom of excess and indulgence— and the very greasy way of life you've been trying so hard to escape.

When you come to your senses a day or week later, you'll feel guilty and perhaps depressed. Maybe, you'll suggest to yourself, you're not cut out for this health and fitness stuff. Maybe you'll never develop the resolve needed to reach your fat reduction goals.

Maybe, you conclude, you should just give up.

Don't do it. Brush the doughnut crumbs from your car seat and move on. Do you stop brushing your teeth because you missed a day? I don't think so. Don't overreact to mistakes or setbacks. You're human. Forgive yourself and get back on track immediately. Focus again on what lies ahead, not on what you're trying to leave behind. The fact is, no one, not even world-class athletes, are at the top of their form every time they step between the white lines. The best basketball players who have ever taken the court missed half their shots; the best hitters in baseball fail almost 70 percent of the time.

Your attitudes, energy levels, and sense of commitment will fluctuate wildly over the course of your fat reduction effort. Far too many novice fat burners expect themselves to be able to push forward continuously. Relax. A smooth cruise to the finish line is probably not going to happen. You may occasionally slip and slide, and you'll find yourself seemingly stuck in neutral from time to time. Don't panic. These plateaus are simply your body and mind's adjustment to new eating and exercise habits. Just when you begin to believe you've stopped improving, you'll find yourself making gains. Perhaps one of my favorite axioms will help you put the ups and downs you're almost certain to experience in perspective: You can't see grass growing, yet it grows nonetheless.

Keep going—day by day, step by step. You can't reverse years of neglect or indifference in a few days. You can't burn thirty pounds of fat without burning six first, and you can't run three miles until you can walk one. Be patient. Your eating and exercise strategies are changing your body's most elemental internal structures. Soon those changes will manifest themselves in your appearance and performance.

If you manage your fat reduction crusade effectively, you'll consistently move forward. As you progress, a certain amount of momentum will build. Until you reach that self-perpetuating stage of the process, remember not to denigrate yourself if you encounter difficulties. Allow yourself not to be perfect. Unrealistic expectations will strain your body and mind, undermine your resolve, and lead to burnout. Try to maintain a relaxed, balanced approach.

The self-assessment tests in Chapter 2 offer an accurate gauge of your rate of progress toward your fat reduction goals. Retake the tests every ten days or so to ensure that you're moving forward rather than drifting away.

Start by keeping a day-by-day account of your eating and exercise patterns over a ten-day period. You may be surprised at what you learn. Is casual simple-carb snacking becoming a regular occurrence? (One dough-nut or one bag of potato chips a day can easily add about thirteen pounds of body fat to your frame in a year.) Are you skipping exercise sessions or not really applying yourself to your body work? Are your meals balanced? Is portion size a problem? A thorough review of your behavior will allow you to answer all those kinds of questions and reveal aspects of your effort that need attention.

Because you spend so much time with them, family members, friends, and colleagues can have a considerable impact on your behavior, attitudes, beliefs, and emotions. Strangely, the people closest to you are also the peo-ple most likely to hinder your fat reduction efforts. Some people who share your life may find the prospect of a new you threatening. Others may become overzealous in their attempts to help and support you, leaving you feeling anxious or pressured. In either case, take charge immediately.

Remind yourself—and anyone else who needs to know—of what you're doing and why. Explain your goals and plans to all those likely to be affect-ed by your fat reduction process, and let everyone know how they can aid or at least not impede your efforts. Your family and friends can be inter-ested, supportive, helpful, cynical, jealous, or pessimistic. Let them say and think what they want. Don't let their attitudes dictate yours. Accept whatever help you get, make whatever accommodations you can meet the needs of others, but remember: It's your body and your life.

If someone close to you becomes seriously interested in your fat reduction strategies, by all means share what you've learned. As an ancient proverb reminds us, we learn best when we teach. Be careful, though. While exercise and eating plans are much easier to carry out when a friend or family member becomes a partner in your efforts, harm-ful competition can sometimes undermine the whole process. If you and your partner view your fat reduction activities as some kind of duel, there could be trouble. Don't become jealous, depressed, or frustrated if your partner seems to be progressing faster than you are. Seeing yourself as "losing" or "falling behind" could alienate you not only from your part-ner but from your own renovation process as well. Be competitive only with yourself. Enjoy your partner's successes and set your own pace to match them.

If your own behavior or attitudes don't explain disappointing assessment test scores and you can't find any significant negative influences exerted by others, it's possible the apparent decline in progress you're experiencing is due to the well-known plateau effect.

At some point in your fat reduction efforts (usually a few weeks to a few months after you begin), your progress may become imperceptible. You have reached a plateau. And while you may not think so, congratulations are in order. You have trained your body to accept (actually, welcome) the demands of your eating and exercise routines. You'll need to provide new challenges to inspire continued improvement. You advanced rapidly at the beginning of your reconstruction process because you had substantial improvement to make. Quick dramatic gains aren't so easy when you're already doing pretty well. Generally, the best way to address the plateau effect is to intensify your workouts and expand your exercise repertoire. You can also try eating variations (see the meal templates in Chapter 8), or add some supplements with your meals as a boost to your metabolism.

Any Questions?

The thousands of fat burners who came before you asked a lot of questions. I hope that my responses to the concerns and issues they raised will prove helpful in your fat reduction campaign.

Q: Is exercise really necessary to lose fat?

A: Yes. Extremely low calorie diets will strip away more muscle and lean tissue than fat. Diet pills and other weight loss drugs can dehydrate you, increase your blood pressure, weaken your heart, and do serious damage to your body and mind.

Q: Is circuit training an effective way to burn fat?

A: My No-Excuses Workout is a form of circuit training, and, yes, it is an extremely efficient method of fat incineration. Conventional resistance training requires rest periods between each set of exercises. The breaks are needed to replenish anaerobic strength levels. In conventional exercise routines, heart rate and blood pressure are elevated only while the exercise is being performed. In circuit training, one exercise immediately follows the other. As is the case in my NEW, exercises are in combinations that isolate single muscles and regional muscle groups. The end result is a total body workout that provides both anaerobic and aerobic benefits.

Q: Should I be applying my exercise with a slow steady pace?

A: Always perform your exercises with control. First learn proper exercise technique; then if you choose, your speeds can improve. However, I have discovered that burning fat is greatly accelerated when short bursts of speed are incorporated into either anaerobic/resistance or aerobic exercise. These short bursts explosively deplete sugar from your bloodstream and muscles forcing your body to shift to burning more fat as fuel. This is what I call Variable Intensity Training, or VIT. (Please refer to illustration on page 127.)

Q: Do those so-called fat-burning products sold today really burn fat? Isn't a strong cup of coffee just as good?

A: Unless you're combining your fat-reduction efforts with regular exercise, you can forget about using any fat-burning product. These products are known to be either ineffective or dangerous to your health, even the OTC brands. Caffeine, however, has always been touted as a great workout stimulant and fat burner, and for good reason. A good cup of coffee is used by plenty of athletes and fitness buffs for the same objectives you're inquiring about. Caffeine from natural sources, in my opinion, is very useful, but please avoid the synthetic sweeteners, fat-laden creams, and other artificial flavor enhancers.

Q: I want to combine my activities and need to know what is better to do first, aerobics or resistance exercise?

A: For fat burning, it is best to perform resistance or anaerobic exercise before your aerobic activity. Resistance training requires more strength and concentration on exercise techniques, as in lifting weights or performing my No-Excuses Workout. Also, since anaerobic exercise utilizes mostly sugars for energy, it is best to deplete your sugar storages so your body can burn more fat during your aerobic activity.

Q: What's the best time of the day to exercise?

A: Early-morning workouts seem to be best for burning fat. In the morning your body's blood sugar level is usually at its lowest point (because you haven't eaten for several hours). With no excess sugars to burn, your body uses fat as the energy source it needs to fuel your early workout. If you are involved in weight training, late afternoon or early evening is a better time to work out. Your body needs the energy you've stored during the day to handle the harsh energy demands of weight work. Also, recent research at Auburn University indicates that your heart and lungs are stronger, your muscles more flexible, and your reactions much faster later in the day.

Q: Sometimes I feel sore after a workout. Should I be concerned?

A: Soreness, at first, is typical, but it will diminish with time. Make sure you are warming up and cooling down properly. Include stretching exercises daily. Review your mechanics and concentrate on your form.

Q: How much time should I spend exercising to become fit?

A: The notion that more is better doesn't really apply when trying to determine how much activity is enough. I firmly believe that you should get as much done in as little time as possible. That's why I designed a seven-minute workout instead of an eighty-seven-minute workout. I encourage my clients to approach their training with vigor, enthusiasm, and focus. However, long, tedious workouts aren't really needed if you know what you're doing and do it correctly. Keep in mind that excessive energy expenditures day after day can weaken the immune system and, through overwork, damage the very internal systems you're trying to improve. As a rule of thumb, three or four sessions a week should be sufficient for most people. It's important to schedule your workouts far enough apart to take advantage of the fat-burning value of the metabolic process. Exercising intensely every day is counterproductive because adequate recuperation time is needed to repair your tissues. If you're involved in strength training, it's essential to limit your workouts to no more than

Variable Intensity Training

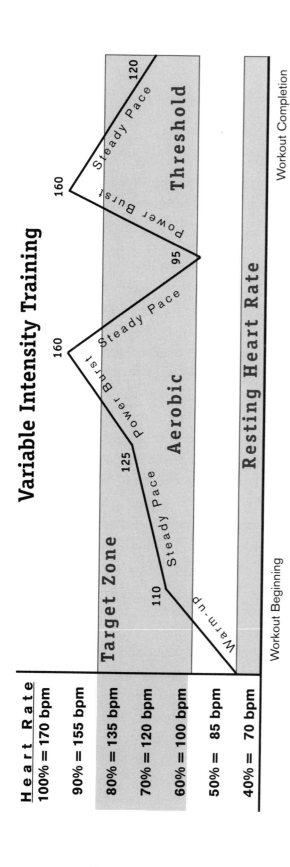

Heart Rate
100% = 170 bpm
90% = 155 bpm
80% = 135 bpm
70% = 120 bpm
60% = 100 bpm
50% = 85 bpm
40% = 70 bpm

Target Zone — Aerobic — Threshold

Warm-up · Steady Pace · Power Burst · Steady Pace · Power Burst · Steady Pace
110 · 125 · 160 · 95 · 160 · 120

Resting Heart Rate

Workout Beginning — Workout Completion

CALCULATION

```
  110
+ 125
+ 160
+  95
+ 160
+ 120
─────
  770
 ÷  6
130 BPM
```

AVERAGE

These illustrations exemplify how a fifty-year-old fitness enthusiast can monitor his/her heart rate with **Variable Intensity Training.** The *Conventional Aerobic Range* (or *Threshold*) suggested for a fifty-year-old is to maintain an intensity between 100–145 bpm. **VIT**, *when averaged out*, enables each applicant to register the proper heart rate (or bpm) throughout the entire workout duration providing excellent fat-burning and health benefits.

BPM = beats per minute.
All figures are rounded.

Heart Rate
100% = 170 bpm
90% = 155 bpm
80% = 135 bpm
70% = 120 bpm
60% = 100 bpm
50% = 85 bpm
40% = 70 bpm

Warm-up 110 · Steady Pace 125 · Power Burst 160 · Steady Pace 95 · Power Burst 160 · Steady Pace 120

Target Zone

four times a week. Overworking muscles can wear out cartilage and cause serious mobility problems as you age.

Q: Can I use laxatives to lose weight?

A: That's not a good idea. Laxatives do nothing to boost your metabolism. In fact, they make it more difficult for your body to absorb food. When you eat correctly and exercise regularly, you also become more regular—if you know what I mean.

Q: What is the value of fiber?

A: Eating fiber causes your body to eliminate rather than store fat. When you consume fiber on a daily basis, your body will absorb fewer calories than if you don't. Fiber also is extremely beneficial for a healthy intestinal tract.

Q: I eat at restaurants several times a week. Can I maintain healthy eating habits?

A: Yes, but remember to eat balanced portions. Choose chicken, fish, or lean beef as a main course. Be wary of menus laced with phrases like breaded, panfried, deep-fried, creamy, au gratin, escalloped, smothered. Request that sauces and dressings be served on the side. Choose a baked potato instead of fries, and you'll avoid a ton of fat. Practice portion control. Most restaurant servings are two or three times as large as they need to be. You can probably take about half your meal home in a doggie bag. And use discretion at the salad bar. A simple green salad and veggies and a low-fat dressing averages about 100 calories and 2 grams of fat. Pile on enough bacon bits and blue cheese dressing, and you'll find yourself in the neighborhood of an extra 700 calories and 30 grams of fat.

Q: I sometimes get headaches after I exercise. Why?

A: You're probably overdoing it. Back off a notch and add a ten-minute cooldown period to your routine. Take a walk or an easy spin on a stationary bike. Reduce your pace gradually until you're breathing regularly. Also, be careful of caffeinated drinks or other hidden chemicals in foods or beverages before exercising.

Q: I do well with my eating plan during the day and at dinner, but I can't seem to avoid snacking at night. How should I adjust my menu?

A: That's easy. Schedule one—and only one—protein snack midway between dinner and bedtime.

Q: Should women lift weights?

A: Weight lifting or some other type of resistance training should be a basic element of everyone's fitness plan. In the long run, weight work is as valuable to women as it is to men. Research indicates that strength training reinforces the musculoskeletal system and slows down the onset of osteoporosis, a bone-thinning condition most commonly found in maturing women. Strength exercise with weights or using your body weight as resistance places a healthy stress on the skeleton and promotes bone growth. Women worried that weight work will make them look like linebackers can relax. A training program such as the NEW that uses multiple reps with light resistance loads and is performed in circuit-training fashion will produce strong bones and lean, firm muscles.

Q: Lately I've been reading a lot about how good aerobic exercise is for my heart and lungs. Can you suggest some simple aerobic activities I can use to supplement my NEW? Keep in mind that I'm not very athletic, and I don't have a lot of money to spend for health club dues.

A: Your NEW does offer aerobic as well as muscle toning benefits. But twenty to forty-five minutes of fitness walking, jogging, or some combination of both on your NEW "off days" should deliver the cardiovascular benefits you're looking for. The only equipment you need is a well-made pair of shoes. If the climate where you live is going to keep you indoors for weeks or months at a time, check to see if any of the gyms in your area offer a "track only" membership that fits your budget or try my "Walk-A-Dobics" routine. If not, don't worry. Visit enough garage, rummage, or yard sales, and you'll eventually find a barely used stationary bike or treadmill that you can afford.

Q: I've acquired a severe case of shinsplints from running. How can I treat this ailment and stay in shape while I'm recuperating?

A: Biking, elliptical stepping, swimming, or rowing will keep you well conditioned while you're unable to run. To treat your shinsplints, I suggest ice massage. Fill a Styrofoam cup with water and freeze it. Once the water's frozen, cut away the top half of the cup, exposing the ice and leaving yourself a convenient Styrofoam grip. Massage your shins in a circular fashion. Apply pressure for deep tissue relief. You can also try a better pair of shoes and a softer surface for a moderately paced walk.

Q: I'm a vegetarian, and I'm concerned that I may not be getting enough protein, vitamins, and minerals from my food. Should I use some sort of vitamin/mineral supplement or one of those protein mixtures?

A: You probably don't need a vitamin or mineral supplement unless you're struggling to summon the energy necessary to exercise properly or you're having trouble recovering from your workouts. Protein can be supplemented quite effectively. There are dozens of products on the market that supply all the essential amino acids that a vegetarian diet may lack. Along with soy, select a protein supplement that can be taken with meals or on an empty stomach. Capsules and powders are best.

Q: What do you consider your most important fitness tip?

A: The idea that I think is essential to get across is that we can all change, and it doesn't take years to do it. Becoming fit and healthy isn't nearly as hard as some people think it is. If you change your behavior just a little bit every day, those small step-by-step changes will soon bring you the body you want.

C H A P T E R **8**

Fun with Food

I love food, and so should you.

I mean real food, of course, not the chemically engineered synthetic dreck that lines so many aisles in our supermarkets. Real food satisfies our body's elemental needs and makes us strong. And real food, selected wisely and prepared creatively, can excite our senses and bring us pleasure, too.

Boredom is the primary reason that restrictive fad diets don't work. The keys to healthy eating are balance and variety. The recipes that follow will show you dozens of tasty, innovative ways to explore and enjoy the fruits, vegetables, grains, meats, fish, and fowl your body wants and needs. As you'll discover, eating wisely doesn't mean you can't eat well.

Healthy cooking requires only a few pieces of equipment and a handful of pantry supplies. A nonstick skillet, which minimizes the need for cooking oil, is essential. If you routinely cook in large quantities, a nonstick Dutch oven would also be helpful. Nonstick cookware with ridges allows fat to drain away from your food as you cook meats over high heat. A rack for roasting or broiling serves the same purpose, as do most of the table-top "grilling machines," such as George Foreman's, that have become popular in the past few years.

The wide range of nonfat, low-fat, and reduced-fat dairy products now routinely available make possible sensible versions of formerly fatty sauces, gravies, and soups. Evaporated skim milk adds noticeable body to soups, stews, and sauces. Buttermilk lends a tangy edge to salad dressing and dumplings. Reduced-fat cheeses work well in a number of dishes.

Fresh herbs and spices add flavor and fragrance to anything you cook. Citrus zest, juices, and vinegar contribute a pleasant sharpness. Used in moderation, salty ingredients such as low-sodium soy sauce, Parmesan cheese, and olives lift flavor levels. Olive oil adds a subtle intensity. Small portions of toasted nuts contribute appealing crunchiness. Onions, garlic, shallots, and scallions provide pungency, and peppers give bland dishes a welcome spark.

As you strive to build your new body, think of your kitchen as your workshop. Be curious and creative. Experiment. And for clever flavorful combinations of high-quality raw materials, try the recipes that follow.

Finally, some of the recipes herein are provided by Jay Robb.

Breakfast

Research indicates that men and women who eat a healthy breakfast every day are less stressed and better able to control body fat levels than those who don't. And, it appears, the healthy breakfast people live longer. Try one or all of the following suggestions.

Bacon and Eggs Lite

A couple of minor substitutions remove most of the grease and fat from this traditional trucker favorite.

5 egg whites
1 egg yolk
2 strips turkey bacon

1 slice whole grain bread

2 teaspoons almond butter or peanut butter

▶ In a lightly oiled nonstick heated skillet, swirl the egg whites and the yoke to cover the pan. Cook sunny side up until the whites are solid and the yoke soft and runny. In another skillet, cook the turkey bacon according to package instructions. Place the cooked bacon on paper towels and pat with a paper towel to remove excess oil. Toast the bread and cover with the almond butter.

The Kitchen Sink Frittata

Use your leftover veggies, lean meat, and chicken to create a quick, interesting start to your day. This can also be used for lunch or dinner.

6 eggs or low-fat egg substitutes

1^{1}/$_{2}$ tablespoons olive oil

2 cups leftover vegetables, meat, fowl, etc., you have handy, cut up

▶ Beat the eggs well and pour into a heated, lightly oiled skillet. After the eggs set firmly (forming sort of a pancake), flip them over. Spoon the leftovers onto one half of the eggs and fold over the other half to cover. Cook until done on each side. Serve with sliced tomatoes or celery sticks. (**Very low carb**)

The Breakfast Mushroom

A mushroom stuffed with fiber for breakfast? Why not. For lunch, too.

8 large fresh mushroom caps

Salt and pepper to taste

4 teaspoons olive oil

1 tablespoon minced garlic

10 ounces fresh spinach leaves, drained and chopped

^{1}/$_{4}$ teaspoon sweet dried basil

1 large green pepper, finely chopped

4 large eggs or egg substitutes

▶ Preheat the oven to 400 degrees. Place the mushroom caps, rounded side down, in a medium glass baking dish. Sprinkle with salt and pepper. Bake until tender, about 12–15 minutes. Remove and place the caps on a plate. Lower the oven temperature to 250 degrees. Place 3 teaspoons of oil in a skillet over medium heat. Add the garlic and sauté until brown, 2–3 minutes. Add the spinach and toss for 2–3 minutes. Stir in the basil. Place the spinach in the baking dish. Add the mushrooms, rounded side down, and fill each cap about halfway with peppers, using half of the peppers. Place the baking dish in the oven to keep the contents warm while you scramble the eggs, using the remaining 1 teaspoon of oil to coat the skillet. Add the scrambled eggs to the mushroom caps and top with the remaining peppers. **(Very low carb)**

Turkey Sausage

Some low-fat, low-carb protein to start your day. Great with eggs!

2 pounds ground turkey

1 tablespoon dried sage

1 tablespoon soy sauce

$1/2$ teaspoon ground pepper

$1/2$ teaspoon dried sweet basil

$1/2$ teaspoon ground cloves

$1/2$ teaspoon nutmeg

1 teaspoon olive oil

▶ Place all the ingredients except the oil in a large bowl and mix well. Divide the mixture into 18–20 equal portions and shape each portion into a patty. Place the oil in a large skillet over moderate heat. Brown the patties on both sides and cook thoroughly. Freeze unused patties for future use. **(Very low carb)**

El Paso Hash

This spicy southwestern-style breakfast works for lunch and dinner, too.

1 tablespoon olive oil
$^1/_2$ cup chopped red bell pepper
$^1/_2$ cup chopped onion
1 large clove garlic, minced
2 cups fully cooked vegetable protein crumbles (12-ounce package)
One 4$^1/_2$-ounce can chopped green chilies
$^1/_4$ teaspoon salt
2 cups, boiled, drained, and diced potatoes (with skin on)
$^1/_4$ cup chopped fresh cilantro

▶ Heat the oil in a large nonstick skillet over medium-high heat. Add the bell pepper, onion, and garlic. Stir and cook until crisp-tender. Stir in the remaining ingredients except the cilantro. Cook 8–10 minutes, or until the potatoes begin to brown. Stir in the cilantro and serve. **(Very low fat)**

The Royal Canadian Frittata

Canadian bacon isn't really bacon; it's actually smoked strips of pork loin, a lean, flavorful meat. You can easily add it to omelets or, in this case, a tasty frittata.

3 eggs
3 tablespoons skim milk
1 teaspoon Dijon mustard
Oil for frying
2 ounces Canadian bacon, chopped ($^1/_2$ cup)
$^1/_4$ cup chopped green bell pepper
$^1/_4$ cup chopped onion
1 small tomato, thinly sliced

1¹/₂ ounces reduced-fat Swiss cheese, shredded

2 teaspoons freshly chopped parsley

▶ Beat the eggs in a mixing bowl. Add the milk and mustard, and mix well. Set aside. Heat a lightly oiled nonstick skillet over medium heat. Add the bacon, bell pepper, and onion. Cook and stir for 4–5 minutes, or until the pepper and onion are crisp-tender. Pour the egg mixture over the bacon mixture. As the eggs cook, tilt the skillet to allow the uncooked egg to flow to the bottom of the skillet. When the eggs are set but the top is still moist, arrange the tomato slices over the top and sprinkle with cheese. Cover the skillet and cook until the cheese is melted. Sprinkle with parsley. Cut the frittata in half or into wedges, slide onto a plate, and serve immediately. **(Very low carb and good protein)**

The Zucchini Frittata

Use firm, fresh zucchini for this breakfast or brunch dish, and you'll be pleasantly surprised by the crisp texture of the open-faced omelet you've created.

3 eggs

¹/₄ cup low-fat cottage cheese

¹/₄ teaspoon salt

¹/₈ teaspoon pepper

Oil for frying

2 small fresh zucchini, thinly sliced

¹/₄ cup chopped red bell pepper

2 tablespoons finely chopped onion

1 tablespoon water

1 ounce reduced-fat Havarti cheese, shredded (¹/₄ cup)

▶ Beat the eggs in a mixing bowl. Add the cottage cheese, salt, and pepper, and mix well. Set aside. Heat a lightly oiled 8-inch skillet over medium-high heat. Add the zucchini, bell pepper, onion, and water. Cook and stir until the vegetables are crisp-tender, about 4–5 minutes. Lower the heat to medium. Pour the egg mixture over the zucchini mixture. As the eggs cook, tilt the skillet to allow the uncooked egg to flow to the bottom of the skillet. When the eggs are set but the top is still moist, sprinkle with cheese. Cover the skillet and cook until the cheese is melted and the eggs are completely set. Cut the frittata in half or into wedges, slide onto a plate, and serve immediately. **(Very low carb)**

Poultry

Once you eliminate their skins, chicken and turkey are pretty much perfect foods. Low in fat and high in protein, poultry pleases our taste buds by absorbing and enhancing all the flavors around it as it cooks. Poultry cooks quickly and contains just enough fat and sugar to brown nicely and contribute deep, rich taste to a variety of low-fat, low-carb sauces.

Spicy Peach Chicken

Any combination of chicken pieces can be used in this recipe, and apricot preserves can be used in place of peach preserves.

1 cup peach preserves
2 tablespoons cider vinegar
$1/2$ teaspoon ginger
$1/4$ cup chopped chilies
6 chicken drumsticks, with skin removed
3 chicken breasts, with skin removed

❭ Combine all the ingredients except the chicken in a food processor or blender and process until smooth. Broil the chicken 4 to 6 inches from the heat source for 25–30 minutes, or until the chicken is fork-tender and the juices run clear. Turn the chicken frequently and brush with the preserves mixture during the last 15 minutes of broiling. **(Very low fat and very low carb)**

Indonesian Chicken

This easy skewer entrée becomes a meal when you add rice and veggies.

2 tablespoons peanut butter
2 tablespoons teriyaki marinade
$1/8$ teaspoon crushed red pepper flakes
1 pound skinless, boneless chicken breast halves, cut into $1/2$-inch-thick strips

▶ Place all the ingredients except the chicken in a small bowl and mix until smooth. Thread the chicken strips onto four 12- to 14-inch skewers. Broil the chicken 4 to 6 inches from the heat source for 8–10 minutes, or until the chicken is no longer pink in the center. Turn the chicken once and baste with the peanut butter sauce. **(Very low fat and almost no carbs at all)**

Herbed Turkey Tenderloins

Turkey tenderloin is extremely lean. Watch closely as you broil them, or they may overcook and dry out.

6 slices bacon
2 (about 12 ounces each) fresh turkey tenderloins
1 tablespoon olive oil
$1/4$ teaspoon pepper
$1/4$ teaspoon dried thyme leaves

▶ Cook the bacon in a skillet for 2–3 minutes per side, or until the bacon begins to brown but is not yet crisp. (The bacon needs to be pliable to wrap around the turkey.) Drain on paper towels. Cut each turkey tenderloin crosswise into 4 pieces. Press the tapered ends of each tenderloin together to form 1 piece. Wrap partially cooked bacon slices around each piece of turkey. Secure with toothpicks. Brush both sides of each piece with the oil. Sprinkle each one with pepper and thyme. Broil 4 to 6 inches from the heat source for 12–15 minutes, or until the bacon is thoroughly browned and crisp. Turn once. Remove the toothpicks before serving. **(Very low fat and not a single carb)**

Turkey Scaloppini

Here's a clever low-fat variation of a traditional Italian dish.

1 pound fresh turkey tenderloin, sliced
$1/2$ teaspoon salt
$1/2$ cup Italian-style bread crumbs
Oil for frying
4 teaspoons margarine or butter
$1/2$ cup dry white wine (such as Chardonnay)
2 tablespoons lemon juice
4–6 lemon slices for garnish
Modest amount of fresh parsley for garnish

▶ Sprinkle the turkey slices with salt and coat on both sides with bread crumbs. Heat a large, lightly oiled nonstick skillet over medium-high heat. Add the turkey and cook for 2–4 minutes, until the turkey is no longer pink. Turn once. Remove the turkey, place on a serving platter, and cover to keep warm. Add the margarine, wine, and lemon juice to the same skillet you used to cook the turkey and bring to a boil. Pour the sauce over the turkey. Garnish with the lemon slices and parsley. **(Very low fat and very low carb)**

Oven-fried Chicken

Fried chicken is made by deep-frying in fat chicken pieces that have been coated with beaten eggs and bread crumbs. This is a healthier way.

2 cups corn flakes, crushed (making 1 cup)
1 egg white

1 teaspoon paprika

¹/₂ teaspoon salt

¹/₂ teaspoon garlic powder

¹/₂ teaspoon dried oregano leaves

¹/₄ teaspoon ground cayenne pepper

One 3–4-pound frying chicken, cut up and skin removed

▶ Heat the oven to 400 degrees. Coat a broiler pan with cooking spray. Place the cereal in a shallow bowl. In another bowl, place the egg white, paprika, salt, garlic powder, oregano, and red pepper. Blend well. Dip the chicken pieces in the mixture and coat with the cereal. (To do this easily, shake the egg-dipped pieces and the cornflakes together in a large plastic food storage bag.) Place the "breaded" chicken on the broiler pan. Bake for 45 minutes, or until the chicken is fork-tender and the juices run clear. **(Very low fat and very low carb)**

Low-Cal Chicken Tacos

Here's a fresh light version of an old classic that offers a tasty way to take advantage of the benefits that avocado provides.

1 boneless, skinless chicken breast

2 corn tortillas

¹/₄ small white onion, chopped

2 cups fresh cilantro, chopped

2 thin slices fresh avocado

2 pounds salsa (fresh is best; store-bought is okay)

▶ Grill the chicken breast and cut it into thin strips. Combine the chicken with the onion, cilantro, avocado, and salsa. Divide the mixture in half. Warm the tortillas using a skillet or microwave, until they are soft. Fill each tortilla with the mixture, roll up, and serve. Add light sour cream, tomatoes, and lettuce if desired.

Skillet Chicken with Mushrooms and Onions

Herbes de Provence is a mixture of basil, fennel seed, marjoram, rosemary, and several other seasonings frequently used in southern France. You can use it not just for this recipe but anytime you want to enhance the flavor of meat, poultry, or vegetables.

$^1\!/_4$ cup whole grain flour

3 teaspoons paprika

Salt to taste

4 boneless, skinless chicken breast halves

1 tablespoon olive oil

$^1\!/_2$ cup dry white wine or chicken broth

1 tablespoon tomato paste

1 teaspoon dried *herbes de Provence*

Two 8-ounce packages fresh mushrooms, sliced (6 cups)

1 cup frozen small white onions, thawed

▶ Place the flour, paprika, and salt in a large resealable plastic food storage bag and mix well. Add the chicken. Shake the bag to coat the chicken with the flour mixture. Heat the oil in a 12-inch nonstick skillet over medium-high heat. Add the coated chicken and cook about 9 minutes, turning the chicken once. Add the wine, tomato paste, and herbs and blend well. Stir in the mushrooms and onions, lower the heat, cover, and simmer for 20–25 minutes, stirring once. Uncover, cook another 3–5 minutes, or until the sauce is slightly thickened.

Turkey Mac

The light Alfredo sauce this recipe calls for can be found next to the refrigerated pasta section of your supermarket.

4 ounces uncooked elbow macaroni (1 cup)

1 pound ground turkey breast

$^3\!/_4$ teaspoon garlic-pepper blend

3 medium zucchini, chopped

2 tablespoons chopped basil leaves

One 10-ounce container light Alfredo sauce

$^1/_4$ cup Italian-style bread crumbs

2 tablespoons grated Romano cheese

1 teaspoon butter or margarine, melted

▸ Heat the oven to 350 degrees. Cook the macaroni according to the package directions, then drain. In a large nonstick skillet, cook and stir the turkey and garlic-pepper blend until the turkey is no longer pink, 6–8 minutes. Add the cooked macaroni, zucchini, basil, and Alfredo sauce, and mix well. Coat a $2^1/_2$-quart casserole dish with cooking spray. Spoon the mixture into the casserole dish. In a small bowl, mix the bread crumbs, cheese, and butter. Sprinkle this mixture over the casserole. Bake for 30–40 minutes, or until thoroughly heated.

Chicken and Vegetable Cacciatore

This dish has a flavorful sauce you're going to love.

1 teaspoon olive oil

4 boneless, skinless chicken breast halves

2 medium carrots, thinly sliced

1 large green, red, or yellow bell pepper, cut into bite-size strips

1 medium onion, chopped

One $14^1/_2$-ounce can tomato sauce with tomato bits and herbs

Chopped parsley for garnish

▸ Heat the oil in a Dutch oven over medium-high heat. Add the chicken, carrots, bell pepper, and onion. Cook for 5 minutes, stirring frequently. Turn the chicken over, add the tomato sauce, and mix well. Turn the heat to low, cover, and simmer for 18–20 minutes, or until the chicken is fork-tender and the juices run clear. Garnish with parsley. **(Very low fat and very low carb)**

Grilled Honey-Tarragon Chicken

This quick, sweet winner shouldn't take more than twenty minutes.

2 tablespoons freshly chopped parsley
2 teaspoons freshly chopped tarragon
Dash of salt
3 tablespoons honey
1 tablespoon lemon juice
4 boneless, skinless chicken breast halves
¼ teaspoon salt
¼ teaspoon pepper

▶ Place the parsley, tarragon, salt, honey, and lemon juice in a small bowl and blend well. Sprinkle the chicken with the salt and pepper. Brush with half of the honey mixture. Broil 4 to 6 inches from the heat source for 8–12 minutes. Turn once and brush with the remaining honey mixture. **(Very low fat and very low carb)**

Pineapple Turkey

Never having been to Hawaii, the Pilgrims would be startled by this interesting combination of flavors.

1 pound fresh turkey tenderloin, cut in half lengthwise
¼ teaspoon salt
⅛ teaspoon pepper
One 6-ounce can pineapple juice (¾ cup)
1 tablespoon chopped green onions
2 teaspoons freshly chopped sage
2 teaspoons freshly chopped thyme

▶ Heat a large, lightly oiled nonstick skillet over medium heat. Sprinkle the turkey with salt and pepper, add to the skillet, cover, and cook for 3 minutes. Turn the turkey, add the pineapple juice, cover, and cook an additional 5–8 minutes, or until the turkey is no longer pink at its center. Remove the turkey from the skillet and place it on a serving platter. Sprinkle with onions, sage, and thyme. Slice and cover with aluminum foil to keep warm. Cook the liquid remaining in the skillet on high heat for 2–3 minutes, or until about $^1/_3$ cup remains. Spoon the liquid over the turkey. **(Almost no fat and very low carb)**

Chicken in Green Sauce

This juicy chicken dish features a healthy herb and pea-flecked sauce, and a dash of hot spice.

1 tablespoon flour
$^1/_2$ teaspoon salt
$^1/_4$ teaspoon freshly ground black pepper
4 skinless, boneless chicken breast halves
2 teaspoons olive oil
1 cup defatted chicken broth
2 cloves garlic, minced
3 tablespoons freshly chopped parsley
2 tablespoons minced chives or scallions
$^1/_2$ teaspoon dried tarragon
$^1/_8$ teaspoon red pepper flakes
1 cup frozen peas

▶ Combine the flour, $^1/_4$ teaspoon salt, and pepper on a plate. Dredge the chicken in the flour mixture, then shake off the excess. Heat the oil in a large nonstick skillet over medium heat. Add the chicken and cook until golden brown, about 5 minutes. Add the remaining ingredients except the peas. Bring to a boil, lower the heat to a simmer, and cook, partially covered, 10 minutes more. Transfer the chicken to a serving plate. Bring the sauce to a boil over medium heat. Add the peas and cook, uncovered, until the sauce is reduced to $^1/_2$ cup, about 3 minutes. Spoon the peas and sauce over the chicken. **(Very low fat and very low carb)**

Spicy Chicken

A rich, tart sauce enlivens this entrée.

1 tablespoon flour
$^1/_2$ teaspoon salt
$^1/_4$ teaspoon ground black pepper
4 skinless, boneless chicken breast halves
2 teaspoons olive oil
12 ounces small red potatoes, diced
$^3/_4$ cup minced scallions
$^1/_3$ cup water
1 cup defatted chicken broth
$^1/_4$ cup thinly sliced gherkins
3 tablespoons ketchup
1 tablespoon Dijon mustard
3 tablespoons freshly chopped parsley
2 tablespoons red wine vinegar

▶ Combine the flour, $^1/_4$ teaspoon salt, and pepper on a plate. Dredge the chicken in the flour mixture, then shake off any excess. Heat the oil in a large nonstick skillet, over medium heat. Add the chicken and cook, turning once, until golden brown, about 5 minutes. Transfer the chicken to a plate. Add the potatoes, scallions, remaining $^1/_4$ teaspoon salt, and water to the pan. Bring to a boil, then lower the heat to a simmer. Cook, covered, stirring occasionally, about 6 minutes. Stir in the broth, gherkins, ketchup, and mustard. Return to a boil and cook, uncovered, for 1 minute. Return the chicken to the skillet lower the heat to a simmer, cover, and cook another 8 minutes. Stir in the parsley and vinegar. **(Very low fat and low carb)**

Parmesan Chicken with Herbed Tomatoes

Aromatic Parmesan cheese adds just the right flavor to this dish.

2 egg whites
1 tablespoon water

$^1/_3$ cup dried bread crumbs

$^1/_4$ cup grated Parmesan cheese

$^1/_4$ teaspoon salt

4 skinless, boneless chicken breast halves

2 teaspoons olive oil

2 tomatoes, cut into 6 slices each

$^3/_4$ teaspoon sugar

$^3/_4$ teaspoon dried oregano

$^1/_4$ teaspoon dried marjoram

▶ Preheat the oven to 400 degrees. Coat a baking sheet with cooking spray. In a shallow dish, beat the egg whites and water until foamy. On a plate, combine the bread crumbs, cheese, and salt. Set aside 2 tablespoons of mixture. Dip the chicken into the egg whites and then into the crumb mixture. Gently press the crumbs into the chicken. Place the chicken on the baking sheet, drizzle with oil, and bake for 12 minutes, or until the chicken is crisp and golden. Arrange the tomatoes on a separate baking sheet and sprinkle with the sugar, oregano, and marjoram. Spoon the 2 reserved tablespoons of crumb mixture on top of the tomatoes. Place the tomatoes in the oven with the chicken and bake for 6–8 minutes, or until the topping is crisp. Place the chicken and tomatoes on plates. **(Very low fat and low carb)**

Fish

Low in fat and high in protein and minerals, fish is rapidly becoming a favorite food of the health-conscious intelligentsia. Using fresh fish as a centerpiece of low-fat, low-carb meals is an excellent strategy, but remember that buying fresh fish requires some care. A well-run fish market will display fresh fish on or under crushed ice. Fillets will be arranged in a single layer in a pan sunk into the ice. Fish should never sit in puddles or smell "fishy."

When buying whole fish, look for bright bulging eyes and bright red gills, and sniff for any foul odors. Make sure that the fish's skin is shiny, not wrinkled or covered with a brownish film. Fillets or fish steaks should look glossy, moist, and intact, as opposed to dry, dull, slimy, or crumbling. When purchasing frozen fish, check the "sell by" date carefully and choose ice-free packages that are frozen solid, not mushy or freezer-burned.

Always store fresh fish in the coldest part of your refrigerator and use it the same day you buy it. If you must freeze fish, wrap it tightly in heavy-duty insulated plastic. Never thaw fish (or any meat or poultry) at room temperature. Use your microwave or refrigerator.

The best way to estimate cooking time for fish is by using the "ten-minute rule." Allow about ten minutes of cooking time for each inch of thickness. A one-and-a-half-inch-thick fillet, for example, will need about fifteen minutes to cook properly. Because fish is so low in fat, it can easily become tough and dry if overcooked, so remove your fish from the heat as soon as it flakes easily when prodded with a fork.

The Easy Breaded Fish Fillet

Any firm white fish that doesn't fall apart just because you look at it will work in this recipe. Choose cod, halibut, flounder, sea bass, or sole. You can't go wrong.

$^3/_4$ cup crushed seasoned croutons
$^1/_4$ cup grated Parmesan cheese
2 teaspoons dried parsley flakes
1 egg
1 tablespoon water
1 tablespoon lemon juice
1 pound fish fillets ($^1/_4$ to $^1/_2$ inch thick)

▶ Heat the oven to 350 degrees. Coat a 10 by 15 by 1-inch baking pan with cooking spray. In a shallow bowl, place the croutons, cheese, parsley, and paprika, and blend well. In another bowl, place the egg, water, and lemon juice, and beat well. Cut the fillets into serving-size pieces. Dip in the egg mixture, then coat with the crouton mixture. Place the fish in the baking pan. Coat with the cooking spray, using it for about 5 seconds. Bake for 10–15 minutes, or until the fish flakes easily with a fork. **(Very low fat and very low carb)**

Salmon Cakes

Red salmon packed in water makes the best cakes. Dress it up with salsa, cocktail sauce, honey mustard, sour cream, and, of course, tartar sauce.

$3/4$ cup bread crumbs
$1/4$ cup finely chopped celery
$1/4$ cup finely chopped onion
$1/4$ cup low-fat sour cream
1 tablespoon Dijon mustard
1 egg white, beaten
One 15-ounce can salmon, drained, deboned, and flaked
One $4^{1}/_{2}$-ounce can chopped green chilies

▶ Place all the ingredients in a large bowl and mix well. Cover and refrigerate for 10 minutes, or until slightly firm. Shape the mixture into 4 patties about $3/4$ inch thick. Coat a 12-inch nonstick skillet with cooking spray and heat over medium-high heat. Add the patties and cook until golden brown, turning once. **(Very low fat and very low carb)**

Peppery Halibut

Halibut is a large ocean fish with firm white flesh that is low in fat and mild in flavor. Here's a quick and easy preparation suggestion.

2 tablespoons flour
$1/2$ teaspoon lemon-pepper seasoning
$1/2$ teaspoon dried parsley flakes
$1/8$ teaspoon garlic powder
Two 6-ounce halibut steaks, about $3/4$ inch thick

▶ In a shallow bowl, place everything except the halibut and mix well. Coat both sides of the halibut with the mixture. Coat a small nonstick skillet with cooking spray. Heat over medium-high heat and add the halibut. Cook for 1–2 minutes on each side, or until brown. Lower the heat to medium and cook for 8–10 minutes, or until the fish flakes easily with a fork. Turn once.

The Light Lively Tuna Melt

For years the tuna melt has been one of our favorite hot sandwiches. This is a light, quick version of the popular classic.

One 9-ounce can water-packed tuna, drained and flaked
$^1/_3$ cup fat-free creamy Caesar salad dressing
2 tablespoons finely chopped green bell pepper
2 tablespoons finely chopped onion
2 Kaiser rolls or English muffins, split
4 slices American cheese

▶ Heat the oven to 350 degrees. In a medium bowl, place the tuna, salad dressing, pepper, and onion and mix well. Spread the tuna mixture evenly on the rolls. Top each half with a cheese slice and place on a cookie sheet. Bake for 15 minutes, or until the cheese is thoroughly melted. **(Very low fat and low carb)**

Meat

Beef and pork, once our primary sources of protein, have fallen into disrepute of late. Both are considered high-fat foods, but if you choose lean cuts of these meats and prepare them wisely, you can obtain the essential nutritional benefits that beef and pork offer without worrying about unhealthy dietary fat levels.

Mighty Meaty Meat Loaf

Here's a beef dish that's high in protein and fiber, and low in fat carbs, sodium, and calories. And it's tasty.

1 1/2 pounds lean ground sirloin
3/4 cup bread crumbs
2 eggs
1 cup chopped white onion
1/2 cup finely chopped green pepper
1/2 cup finely chopped celery
2 tomatoes, chopped
1/2 cup fresh cilantro, stems removed
Small piece of fresh ginger, peeled and grated

▶ Heat the oven to 325 degrees. In a bowl, mix the ground sirloin, bread crumbs, eggs, onion, green pepper, celery, and one chopped tomato. Shape the mixture into a loaf, place in a nonstick baking dish, and bake for 1 hour. Remove from the oven and let cool. Top with the remaining chopped tomato, cilantro, and ginger.

Pizza Omelet Supreme

This quick change-of-pace meal works well for lunch, brunch, or dinner.

2 ounces lean ground sirloin
2 eggs, beaten
1 teaspoon olive oil
1 tablespoon pizza sauce
1 ounce mozzarella cheese
1/8 white onion, diced
3 black olives, thinly sliced

▶ In a lightly oiled medium skillet, cook the ground sirloin and onion. Set aside. Place the oil in a separate pan and heat over medium heat. Add the eggs and tilt the pan until the eggs cover the bottom of the pan. Cook until the eggs are firm, about 1–2 minutes. Slide the cooked eggs onto a plate and cover with pizza sauce and the ground sirloin and onion. Top with cheese and olives. If you prefer melted cheese, slip the omelet into the microwave for about 20 seconds.

Panfried Steak with Mustard Sauce

Despite their small size, beef tenderloin steaks are very satisfying—rich, tender, and flavorful.

Four 4-ounce beef tenderloin steaks, 1 inch thick
2 teaspoons coarse-ground black pepper
2 cloves garlic, minced
$^1/_3$ cup dry red wine
$^1/_3$ cup beef broth
1 tablespoon Dijon mustard

▶ Coat both sides of the steaks with pepper. Coat a medium skillet with cooking spray and heat over medium-high heat until it is hot. Add the steaks and cook for 6–12 minutes, or until done to your preference. Turn once. Add the garlic, cook, and stir for 1 minute. Add the wine and broth. Cook 1 minute more. Remove the steaks from the skillet and cover to keep warm. Using a wire whisk, stir the mustard into the pan until it is well blended. Serve the sauce over the steaks. **(Low fat and very low carb)**

Apple and Onion Pork Chops

You can use any all-purpose apple for this quick and easy main dish, but recently picked local apples will provide the richest flavor.

4 boneless pork loin chops
$^1/_4$ teaspoon crushed dried thyme leaves
$^1/_8$ teaspoon salt
$^1/_8$ teaspoon pepper

1 teaspoon olive oil

2 medium cooking apples, thinly sliced

1 medium onion, sliced

2 tablespoons brown sugar

2 teaspoons apple cider vinegar

▶ Sprinkle the pork chops with thyme, salt, and pepper. Heat the oil in a large nonstick skillet over medium-high heat. Add the pork chops, cover, and cook for 3 minutes. Turn the chops. Cover and cook 3–5 minutes more, or until the pork is no longer pink at its center. Remove the chops from the skillet and cover to keep warm. Add the apples, onions, and sugar to the same skillet, mix well, and cover. Cook over medium-high heat for 5 minutes, stirring once. Add the vinegar and cook, uncovered, for 3–6 minutes, or until the apples and onion are tender and light golden brown. Serve the apple mixture with the pork chops. **(Low fat and very low carb)**

Slow-Cooked Barbecued Beef Sandwiches

This recipe is enough for twenty sandwiches. That's because this slowly cooked meat is perfect for freezing. If you pack the barbecued beef into pint-sized airtight containers immediately after cooking, you can safely store this tasty treat for up to three months.

3 to 4 pounds lean round steak, trimmed of fat and cut into 1-inch pieces

1 cup finely chopped onions

$^1/_2$ cup firmly packed brown sugar

1 tablespoon chili powder

$^1/_2$ cup ketchup

$^1/_3$ cup cider vinegar

One 12-ounce can light beer

One 6-ounce can tomato paste

▶ In a 3- to 4-quart slow cooker, combine all the ingredients and cover. Cook on low for 10–12 hours. Using a slotted spoon, remove the beef from the sauce and place in a large bowl. Place the sauce in a separate large bowl. Use two large forks to pull apart and shred the beef. Add 2 cups of the sauce.

Spoon the mixture onto whole grain sandwich buns. **(Low fat and low carb)**

T-bone Steak with Mushroom Sauce

This hearty Window of Opportunity Meal entrée can also be made with a mixture of bottled steak sauce, lemon, and pineapple juice.

1 clove garlic, minced
3 tablespoons favorite steak sauce (A-1, Heinz 57, etc.)
Two 1-pound T-bone steaks
^{1}/3 cup beef broth
One 4^1/2-ounce jar mushrooms, drained and liquid reserved
2 teaspoons cornstarch
2 teaspoons freshly chopped parsley

▶ Heat a grill or broiler. Combine the garlic and 1 tablespoon of steak sauce in a small bowl. Set aside. Add enough broth to the reserved mushroom liquid to make ^{3}/4 cup. In a small saucepan, place the remaining 2 tablespoons of steak sauce, broth mixture, mushrooms, and cornstarch, and mix well. Bring to a boil over medium heat and boil for 1 minute, stirring occasionally. Remove from the heat. Stir in the parsley and cover to keep warm. Place the steaks on the grill or broiler 4 to 6 inches from the heat source. Brush with garlic and steak sauce mixture. Cook for 7–12 minutes, or until the steak is done to your liking. Turn once. Serve the steaks topped with the mushroom sauce. **(Very low carb and moderate fat)**

Pork and Rice Skillet

Today's lean pork cooks quickly—which explains how this dish can be ready to eat in about thirty-five minutes.

Four 4-ounce boneless center-cut pork chops, about $1/2$ inch thick

$1/4$ teaspoon salt

Dash of pepper

One 6.7-ounce package brown or wild rice with mushrooms mixture

2 cups water

1 large tomato, cut into 4 slices and halved crosswise

1 large onion, cut into 4 slices and halved crosswise

$1/2$ cup freshly chopped parsley plus 2 tablespoons

▶ Coat a large skillet with cooking spray. Heat over high heat until the pan is very hot. Sprinkle the pork chops with salt and pepper. Place the chops in the skillet and cook 1 minute. Remove the skillet from the heat, and remove the chops from the skillet. Set aside. In the same skillet, combine the rice mixture and seasoning packet with water, and mix well. Arrange alternating slices of tomato and onion in a single layer over the rice mixture. Sprinkle on $1/2$ cup parsley. Arrange the pork chops on top and bring to a boil. Lower the heat to medium, cover tightly, and simmer about 25 minutes, until the pork is no longer pink at its center. Remove the skillet from the heat. Sprinkle on 2 tablespoons parsley. Let stand for 5 minutes before serving. **(Low fat and Low carb)**

Braised Swiss Steak

Top round steak is low in fat, which is the reason it isn't usually very tender. Cooking the steak in a small amount of liquid corrects that problem nicely.

2 cups sliced onions

2 teaspoons condensed beef broth

$1/4$ teaspoon pepper

Two 14-ounce cans diced tomatoes (don't drain)

$1/2$ cup water

$1^1/2$ pounds top round steak

▶ In a Dutch oven or a 12-inch skillet, place all the ingredients except the steak and mix well. Place the steak on top and bring to a boil, stirring gently. Lower the heat, cover, and simmer 1½–2 hours, or until the steak is tender. (**Very low fat and very low carb**)

Southwest Herb Flank Steak

This easy recipe brings zest and flavor to an extremely lean cut of beef.

1 pound flank steak
1 cup chopped Italian plum tomatoes (4 to 6 tomatoes)
¼ cup lime juice
3 tablespoons freshly chopped cilantro
1 tablespoon freshly chopped oregano
¼ teaspoon salt

▶ Score the steak on both sides. Place it in a resealable plastic food storage bag. Place the remaining ingredients in a bowl and mix well. Spoon the mixture over the steak in the bag, seal the bag, and let marinate for 15 minutes. Coat a broiler pan with nonstick cooking spray. Place the steak in the pan and brush with marinade, reserving the remainder. Broil the steak 4 to 6 inches from the heat source for 10–15 minutes, or until the steak is done to your liking. Turn once. Using a slotted spoon, remove the tomatoes from the marinade and spread on the steak. Broil 3–5 minutes more, until the tomatoes are lightly browned. To serve, cut the steak diagonally across the grain into thin slices. (**Very low fat and almost no carbs**)

Strive for Five

Over 150 studies of diverse populations in seventeen different countries have validated the positive effects of a diet rich in fruits and vegetables. The more of these cancer fighters we can fit into our eating strategy, the better off we will be. The U.S. Department of Agriculture recommends at least five servings of fruits and vegetables a day.

Five a day sounds like a challenge until we realize that we have all day to reach that goal and, as the recipes in this section prove, lots of tasty options to reach our goal. In addition to these specific meal and snack suggestions, we can make small adjustments to our everyday eating habits to include more fruits and vegetables in our daily fare, such as:

- adding alfalfa bean sprouts, or shredded carrots to sandwiches
- adding mashed boiled turnips or parsnips into mashed potatoes
- adding shredded fresh spinach or parsley to soups, stews, and omelets
- adding beans, corn, or diced beets to tossed green salads
- serving tuna, egg, or chicken salad in a hollowed-out tomato or a bed of lettuce instead of on bread
- adding raw carrots, celery, or sugar snap peas to our snack menus
- topping cereal with berries or other fruit
- adding frozen peas and corn to canned soups

Grilled Eggplant Parmesan

This easy main dish features an interesting vegetable in a tasty sauce. Use firm, smooth-skinned eggplants with no blemishes or soft spots.

1 medium red onion, cut into 8 wedges
One 1 pound eggplant, cut crosswise into 8 slices
$1/4$ teaspoon salt
$1/8$ teaspoon pepper
One 14-ounce jar meatless spaghetti sauce
4 ounces mozzarella cheese, shredded (1 cup)
$1/4$ cup grated Parmesan cheese

▶ Heat a grill. Thread onion wedges onto a 12- to 14-inch skewer. Coat the onion wedges and eggplant slices with cooking spray. Sprinkle with salt and pepper, and place on the grill 4 to 6 inches from medium-high heat. Cook for 8–10 minutes, or until tender, turning once. Coat a disposable 12- by 8-inch foil pan with cooking spray. Spread $1/2$ cup spaghetti sauce in the bottom of the pan. Arrange the grilled eggplant slices on the sauce. Top with the remaining spaghetti sauce, grilled onion, mozzarella, and Parmesan. Place the pan on the grill and cover loosely with foil. Cook for 3–5 minutes, or until the sauce is bubbly and the cheese is melted. **(Low fat and very low carb)**

Twice-Baked Squash

The best buttercup squash is round and squat, with a turbanlike top. You can also use acorn or golden acorn squash in this recipe.

3 small buttercup squash (about 2 pounds)
$^1/_3$ cup low-fat sour cream
$^1/_2$ teaspoon salt
$^1/_4$ teaspoons nutmeg
6 tablespoons brown sugar

▶ Heat oven to 425 degrees. Cut the squash in half lengthwise. Scoop out and discard the seeds. Place the squash in an ungreased 13- by 9-inch (3-quart) baking dish and cover tightly with foil. Bake at 425 degrees for 30–40 minutes, or until the squash is tender. Cool for 10 minutes. Lower the oven temperature to 375 degrees. Scoop out the squash into a medium mixing bowl, leaving a $^1/_4$-inch-thick shell. Set aside the shells. Add the sour cream, salt, and nutmeg to the squash and mix until smooth. Fill the shells with the squash mixture. Sprinkle each shell with 1 tablespoon of brown sugar. Place the filled shells in the baking dish and bake for 15–20 minutes. **(Very low carb and no fat at all)**

Peach and Pecan Cornbread Dressing

Dried apples or apricots can be used instead of peaches in this dressing.

$1^1/_4$ cups water
1 cup chicken broth

One 8-ounce package cornbread stuffing mix

1 cup chopped celery

$1/2$ cup cut-up dried peaches

$1/4$ cup chopped pecans

▶ Heat the oven to 375 degrees. Coat a 2-quart casserole dish with cooking spray. In a large saucepan, bring water to a boil, stir in all the ingredients, and mix well. Spoon the dressing into the casserole dish, cover, and bake for 20–25 minutes, or until thoroughly heated. **(Very low fat and low carb)**

Beans and Nuts

This is the easiest and best-tasting way I can think of to combine two very healthy foods.

1 package frozen green beans

Handful of almonds, peanuts, or cashews

▶ Cook the green beans according to the package directions. Stir in the nuts.

Grilled Cheesy Tomatoes

Shredded mozzarella or string cheese can be used instead of blue cheese in this recipe.

2 large tomatoes

$1/3$ cup crumbled blue cheese

1 tablespoon olive oil

1 tablespoon freshly chopped basil

2 tablespoons grated Parmesan cheese

▶ Cut the tomatoes in half crosswise. With a small spoon or a melon baller, scoop out the seeds from the tomatoes. Fill the cavities with the blue cheese. Drizzle the tomatoes with the oil. Sprinkle with the basil and

Parmesan. Place the tomatoes, cut side up, on heavy-duty aluminum foil or in a disposable foil pan. Broil about 4 to 6 inches from the heat source for 15 minutes, or until the tomatoes begin to soften. **(Low fat and very low carb)**

Sweet Potato and Apple Toss

This sweet and savory side dish is full of vitamin A.

2 medium apples, quartered and cored
1 large sweet potato (12 ounces), peeled and cut up
$^1/_8$ teaspoon salt
$^1/_8$ teaspoon pepper
1 teaspoon olive oil
$^1/_4$ cup water

▶ In a large bowl, mix together the apples, sweet potato, salt, and pepper. Heat the oil in a skillet over medium heat. Add the apple-potato mixture and water. Cook for 13–18 minutes, or until the sweet potato pieces are tender. Turn the mixture over occasionally. **(Very low fat and low carb)**

Vegetable Curry with Rice

Adding a 15-ounce can of garbanzo beans to this spicy creation increases both fiber and protein.

1 cup uncooked long-grain rice
$3^3/_4$ cups water
2 tablespoons flour
1 tablespoon olive oil
3 teaspoons curry powder
$^1/_2$ teaspoon salt
$^1/_4$ teaspoon cumin
Dash of cayenne pepper

1 small onion, coarsely chopped

1 clove garlic, minced

6 small new potatoes, cut into 1-inch cubes

2 medium carrots, cut into 1-inch pieces

1 extra-large vegetable bouillon cube

2 cups small broccoli florets

2 cups small cauliflower florets

$1/2$ red bell pepper, chopped

▶ Cook the rice in 2 cups of water according to the package directions. Combine $1/4$ cup of water and flour in a small bowl. Beat with a wire whisk until smooth, then set aside. Heat the oil in a large saucepan over medium-high heat. Add the curry powder, salt, cumin, and cayenne pepper. Cook and stir for 1 minute. Add the onion and garlic. Cook and stir 1 minute more. Add the potatoes, carrots, bouillon cube, and remaining $1^{1}/2$ cups of water. Bring to a boil, lower the heat, cover, and simmer for 10 minutes. Add the broccoli, cauliflower, and bell pepper. Cover and simmer for 4–6 minutes, or until the vegetables are tender. Stir the flour mixture into the saucepan. Cover and cook over medium heat, stirring constantly, until the mixture boils and thickens. Serve over the rice. **(Very low fat and moderate carbs)**

Pepper Pasta with Pesto

Penne pasta can be used instead of ziti in this recipe.

8 ounces (2 cups) uncooked ziti

1 tablespoon olive oil

1 medium onion, cut into thin wedges

1 medium red bell pepper, cut into bite-size strips

1 medium yellow bell pepper, cut into bite-size strips

1 small green bell pepper, cut into bite-size strips

$1/3$ cup pesto (you can buy this in a supermarket)

2 teaspoons balsamic vinegar

Salt and pepper to taste

1 ounce Parmesan cheese, shredded ($^1/_4$ cup)

▶ Cook the ziti according to the package directions. Heat the oil in a 12-inch skillet over medium-high heat. Stir in the onion and cook for 2 minutes. Stir in the bell peppers and cook for 3–5 minutes, or until the onion and peppers are crispy-tender. Add the cooked ziti and stir gently to mix. Remove from the heat and stir in the pesto and vinegar. Add the salt and pepper, and sprinkle with cheese.

Bean Patties

You won't believe how tasty these little veggie cakes are.

One 15-ounce can cannellini beans, drained and rinsed
1 tablespoon lemon juice
1 egg
$^1/_3$ cup Italian-style bread crumbs
2 tablespoons grated Parmesan cheese
$^1/_2$ plum tomato, chopped
2 tablespoons finely chopped celery
2 tablespoons finely chopped green bell pepper
2 tablespoons finely chopped onion
$^1/_4$ teaspoon garlic salt
$^1/_4$ teaspoon hot pepper sauce
2 tablespoons tartar sauce

▶ Mash the beans in a medium bowl. Add the lemon juice and egg and blend well. Add the remaining ingredients except the tartar sauce and mix well. Shape into three 4-inch patties. Coat a skillet with cooking spray and heat over medium-high heat. Using a spatula, transfer the patties to the skillet. Cook for 6–8 minutes, or until lightly browned, turning once. Top each patty with about 2 teaspoons of tartar sauce. **(Very low fat and low carb)**

Salad Daze

If you still think of salad as a wedge of rusty lettuce drenched in thick Thousand Island lava, think again. Crunchy, colorful, creative salads are essential allies as we strive to consume five servings of fruit and vegetables every day. In fact, as you'll see when you scan the following recipes, the addition of simply prepared protein can make a salad a meal.

Remember that your Window of Opportunity Meal must include a salad—but not necessarily the same salad every day.

Fresh Fruit Fiesta

Choose organic fruit for this salad, and the tasty side dish will deliver bonus vitamins and minerals.

1 red Delicious apple, cored, peeled, and cut into 1-inch pieces
$1/2$ cup blueberries (fresh if you can get them, frozen if not)
12 seedless grapes
1 navel orange, peeled and sectioned, with sections cut in half
1 peach, pitted, peeled, and cut into bite-size pieces
1 navel orange, peeled and cut into 6 round slices

▶ Place half the blueberries and all the grapes, orange sections, and peach and apple pieces in a large serving bowl. Toss lightly. Arrange the round orange slices in a ring on top. Add the remaining blueberries in the center of the ring. **(Almost no fat and moderate carbs)**

Tangy Waldorf Salad

The Waldorf salad was created in 1893 to celebrate the opening of the hotel for which it is named. In this version of that classic, a snappy vinaigrette replaces the high-fat mayonnaise found in the original.

2 tablespoons olive oil

1 tablespoon red wine vinegar

1 teaspoon sugar

$^1/_2$ teaspoon Dijon mustard

$^1/_8$ teaspoon pepper

2 cups finely chopped apples

1 cup finely chopped celery

2 tablespoons raisins

3 cups mixed salad greens (packaged, if you like)

▸ Combine the oil, vinegar, sugar, mustard, and pepper in a small jar with a tight-fitting lid. Shake well. In a large bowl, combine the apples, celery, and raisins. Pour the vinaigrette over this apple mixture and toss gently. Cover and refrigerate at least 1 hour before serving. To serve, divide the salad greens evenly and spoon the apple mixture over the greens. **(Very low fat and very low carb)**

Island Egg Salad

This salad is high in protein, low in fat, low in carbs, and high in fiber. And fresh pineapple contains the enzyme bromelain, a naturally occurring substance that aids in the digestion of protein.

2 hard-boiled eggs, peeled

1 green onion, chopped

1 stalk celery, washed and finely chopped, plus 6 stalks

1 sprig fresh dill, chopped

1 tablespoon Dijon mustard

3 tablespoons plain nonfat yogurt

1 slice fresh pineapple, chopped

Black pepper to taste

▸ Place the eggs, onion, 1 stalk celery, dill, mustard, yogurt, and pineapple in a bowl and mix well. Fill the 6 celery stalks with the mixture. Dust lightly with black pepper. **(Very low fat and very low carbs)**

The Lean Green Bean Salad

This spicy, crunchy salad makes simple grilled chicken a tasty no-fuss meal.

2 cups green beans, steamed until tender
4 ounces grilled chicken breast, cut into bite-size pieces
1 carrot, grated
1 radish, grated
1/4 red onion, chopped
2 teaspoons mustard powder
8 cherry tomatoes
1 tablespoon Annie's Green Goddess dressing

▶ Place the green beans in 1 layer on a serving plate and spread evenly. Top with the chicken, carrot, radish, onion, mustard, tomatoes, and dressing.

Garden Salad with Herbed Vinaigrette

Fresh herbs dress up and enliven this classic side salad.

1/3 cup chopped basil
3 tablespoons freshly chopped chives
2 tablespoons sugar
1 teaspoon dried mustard
3/4 teaspoon salt
3/4 teaspoon pepper
1/3 cup white wine vinegar
1/2 cup extra-virgin olive oil
One 10-ounce package romaine-blend salad greens

One 8-ounce package sliced fresh mushrooms

1 cup sliced radishes

2 large tomatoes, chopped

▶ Place the basil, chives, sugar, mustard, salt, pepper, vinegar, and oil in a small bowl or a jar with a tight-fitting lid. Blend or shake until the sugar is dissolved. Combine the salad greens, mushrooms, radishes, and tomatoes in a large serving bowl. Add the vinaigrette mixture, toss gently, and serve immediately. **(Very low fat and very low carb)**

Pepper Steak Salad

Wondering what to do with leftover roast beef? Use it in this salad. Chinese (or Napa) cabbage is crunchy and mild, but if you prefer, use coleslaw mix in its place.

$^1/_4$ cup olive oil

3 tablespoons red wine vinegar

2 tablespoons Dijon mustard

1 tablespoon soy sauce

$^1/_4$ teaspoon pepper

1 clove garlic, minced

2 cups shredded Chinese (Napa) cabbage

8 ounces cooked lean roast beef, cut into strips or chunks

1 cup halved cherry tomatoes

1 cup freshly sliced mushrooms

$^1/_2$ cup sliced celery

$^1/_2$ large green bell pepper, cut into bite-size strips

▶ Combine the oil, vinegar, mustard, soy sauce, pepper, and garlic in a small bowl or a jar with a tight-fitting lid. Mix well. Combine the cabbage, beef, tomatoes, mushrooms, celery, and bell pepper in a large serving bowl. Pour the dressing over the salad, toss gently, and serve immediately. **(Very low carb and low fat)**

Tuna Steak Salad

This isn't coffee shop tuna salad—it's much tastier and far more satisfying.

8 ounces tuna steaks
1 teaspoon olive oil
1 small clove garlic, minced
3 large Italian plum tomatoes, sliced lengthwise
4 ounces mozzarella cheese, sliced
2 tablespoons balsamic vinaigrette
2 tablespoons chopped fresh basil

▶ Heat a grill or broiler. Drizzle both sides of the tuna steaks with oil. Rub with the garlic. Let stand at room temperature for 15 minutes to marinate. Arrange the tomato slices around the outer edge of a large serving plate. Arrange the cheese slices inside the ring of tomatoes, overlapping the tomatoes slightly. Drizzle with the vinaigrette and sprinkle with basil. Set aside. Grill or broil the tuna 4 to 6 inches from the heat source. Cook for 8–10 minutes, or until the tuna flakes easily with a fork. Do not turn. Flake the tuna into chunks. Arrange the chunks in the center of the tomatoes and cheese on the platter. **(Low fat and very low carb)**

Soups, Side Dishes, and Snacks

Our need for variety and sensory stimulation in the foods we eat is best satisfied by an eating plan that includes—or, better yet, encourages—a wide range of complementary dishes. Soups and snacks offer quick, easy nourishment when we have neither the time nor the appetite for a full-fledged meal.

Spicy Super Soup

This satisfying soup is rich in vitamins, minerals, and fiber. By adding protein and a salad you create a complete meal.

2 cups water

$^1/_2$ red bell pepper, chopped

1 large red onion, chopped

1 tablespoon olive oil

1 carrot, thinly sliced

2 cups coarsely chopped green cabbage

1 tomato, chopped

2 stalks celery, chopped

1 small piece fresh ginger, peeled and finely sliced

1 tablespoon chili powder

1 tablespoon parsley flakes

1 tablespoon dulse flakes

▶ In a large soup kettle, bring the water to a boil. Add the vegetables and seasonings, and bring the water to a boil again. Lower the heat and simmer for 15–25 minutes, or until the vegetables are crisp-tender. **(Low fat and low carb)**

Southern Gumbo

Hot pepper sauce adds spice to a soup that has been around since the Louisiana Purchase.

1 teaspoon olive oil

1 cup chopped onions

2 cloves garlic, minced

1 cup chopped celery

1 medium green bell pepper, chopped

8 ounces boneless pork loin, cut into thin strips

$2^1/_2$ cups chicken broth

$^1/_2$ teaspoon dried thyme leaves

$^1/_2$ teaspoon dried basil leaves

$^1/_2$ to 1 teaspoon hot pepper sauce

One 14¹/₂-ounce can diced tomatoes (with their juice)

1 cup uncooked instant rice

One 12-ounce package frozen cooked, shelled and deveined, shrimp, thawed

▶ Heat the oil in a Dutch oven over medium-high heat. Add the onions, garlic, celery, and peppers. Cook and stir for 5 minutes. Add the pork and cook for 2–3 minutes, or until the pork is no longer pink. Add the broth, thyme, basil, hot pepper sauce, and tomatoes, and mix well. Bring to a boil. Stir in the rice and shrimp. Remove from the heat and let stand 5 minutes, or until the shrimp are hot. (**Low fat and low carb**)

Creamy Garlic Mashed Potatoes

The Egyptian slaves who built the pyramids ate garlic because they believed it gave them strength. Today we use garlic in recipes like this one because we know it gives us flavor.

4 medium russet or baking potatoes, peeled and cut into quarters

1 small head garlic, separated into cloves and peeled

Water

¹/₂ teaspoon salt

¹/₂ teaspoon pepper

¹/₃ cup heated skim milk

¹/₄ cup light sour cream

▶ Place the potatoes and garlic in a medium saucepan and add enough water to cover. Bring to a boil, then lower the heat to medium-low. Cover loosely and boil gently for 15–20 minutes, or until the potatoes break apart easily when pierced with a fork. Drain well. Mash the potatoes and garlic until no lumps remain. Add the remaining ingredients and continue mashing until the potatoes are smooth. (**Extremely low fat and low carb**)

Turkey Wrap

Here's a guilt-free high-fiber snack that takes maybe three minutes to pre-pare. This recipe is for one person.

$1/2$ tablespoon almond butter or whipped peanut butter
2 stalks celery, washed and halved
2 ounces thinly sliced turkey breast

▶ Spread the almond butter evenly in the convenient little trench of the celery stalk. Wrap the filled celery in a turkey slice. Eat. If you find some cherry tomatoes and baby carrots in the refrigerator, eat them, too. **(Low fat and low carb)**

Turkey Wrap II

Meet the son of Turkey Wrap—even easier to put together than the origi-nal and just as healthy. This recipe is for one person.

2 links string cheese
2 thin slices turkey breast

▶ Roll the string cheese up in the turkey. Eat. Add celery or raw carrots if you crave crunch.

Hot and Cheesy Spinach Delight

This snack's name pretty much says it all.

1 8-ounce package low-fat cream cheese, softened
1 10-ounce package frozen creamed spinach, thawed
7 to 8 ounces Swiss cheese, shredded
1 teaspoon garlic powder
1 loaf French bread

▶ Heat the oven to 350 degrees. In a medium bowl, beat the cream cheese until smooth. Add the spinach, cheese, and garlic powder. Cut a 1-inch V in the top of the bread loaf.

Remove the resulting wedge and discard. Using a spoon, spread the spinach mix into the bread. Wrap securely in foil and bake for 10 minutes, or until thoroughly heated. Cut into slices to serve. **(Low fat and low carb)**

Apricot Trail Mix

Here's a tasty, crunchy snack that is rich in fiber and low in fat.

3 tablespoons honey
$3/4$ teaspoon pumpkin pie spice
1 teaspoon water
1 cup Rice Chex cereal
1 cup low-fat granola cereal
1 cup fat-free pretzels, broken into small pieces
One 6-ounce package chopped dried apricots
$1/2$ cup dried fruit bits

▶ Heat the oven to 325 degrees. Lightly coat a 15- by 10-inch baking pan with cooking spray. Combine the honey, pumpkin pie spice, and water in a small bowl. Set aside. In a large bowl, combine the cereals and pretzel pieces. Coat lightly with the cooking spray and toss once or twice. Stir in all the dried fruit. Drizzle the honey mixture over the cereal mixture and toss gently. Spread evenly in the prepared pan. Bake until the cereal is toasted, stirring occasionally. Cool for 15 minutes. **(Very low fat and low carb)**

Guacamole

Avocados are rich in monounsaturated fat and low in cholesterol. They're also an excellent source of potassium and dietary fiber.

2 ripe avocados, skinned and pitted
$1/2$ cup nonfat or low-fat plain yogurt
$1/2$ cup fresh cilantro leaves, washed and stems removed
Juice of 1 fresh lime

1 small ripe tomato, chopped

$1/2$ small white onion, chopped

▶ In a mixing bowl, mash the avocados with a fork. Add the yogurt and continue mashing until the mixture is creamy smooth. Add the remaining ingredients and mix until well blended. Use baked corn tortilla chips, rice crackers, cucumber slices, or celery for dipping.

The No-Bacon BLT

Bacon-flavored vegetable protein bits are made from wheat and soybeans. They can be found in the salad dressing aisle of your supermarket.

$1/4$ cup low-fat ranch dressing

2 tablespoons bacon-flavored vegetable protein bits

8 slices whole grain bread, toasted

4 lettuce leaves

1 avocado, pitted, peeled, and sliced

1 large tomato, sliced

▶ Place the ranch dressing and protein bits in a small bowl and mix well. Spread the mixture evenly over 4 slices of the toasted bread. Layer the lettuce, avocado, and tomato over the salad dressing mixture. Top with the remaining bread slices. **(High "good" fat and low carb)**

Pizza Quick

This convenient snack satisfies your need for pizza immediately.

2 slices whole grain bread, toasted

4 tablespoons your favorite pasta sauce

2 ounces mozzarella cheese, sliced or shredded

▶ Place the toast on a plate or cookie sheet and top evenly with the pasta sauce and cheese. Place in a toaster oven or broiler. Cook for a few minutes, until the cheese melts. Add mushrooms and green peppers if you like.

Jack Cheese Taters

Monterey Jack is a mild, moist cheese that works well in cooked dishes.

4 medium russet or baking potatoes, peeled and cut into quarters
$1/2$ teaspoon salt
$1/8$ teaspoon pepper
$1/2$ cup heated skim milk
2 ounces hot pepper Monterey Jack cheese, shredded
$1/2$ cup chopped fresh tomato

▶ Place the potatoes in a medium saucepan and add enough water to cover. Bring to a boil, lower the heat to medium-low, cover loosely, and cook for 15–20 minutes, or until the potatoes break apart easily when pierced with a fork. Drain well. Mash the potatoes until the lumps are gone. Add the salt, pepper, and milk, and continue mashing until the potatoes are smooth. Spoon the potatoes into a serving bowl and top with cheese and tomato. **(Low fat and low carb)**

Tomato-Zucchini Salsa on Melba Toast

Crunch and spice come together in this satisfying veggie snack.

2 medium tomatoes, chopped
$1/2$ cup finely chopped zucchini
$1/2$ cup finely chopped green bell pepper
$1/4$ cup sliced ripe olives
2 tablespoons freshly chopped basil
$1/4$ teaspoon garlic powder
32 melba toast rounds or baked tortilla chips

▶ Place all the ingredients except the melba toast in a medium bowl and mix well. To serve, top each toast round with about 1 tablespoon of vegetable mixture. **(Very low fat and low carb)**

Honey Dijon Deviled Eggs

If you like deviled eggs, try this classy version.

7 large hard-boiled eggs
$^1\!/_4$ cup honey Dijon salad dressing
2 tablespoons finely chopped green onions
$^1\!/_8$ teaspoon pepper (optional)

▶ Carefully cut the shelled eggs in half. Remove the yolks, place in a small bowl, and mash with a fork. Add the salad dressing and onions, and mix well. Spoon the mixture into the egg white halves and sprinkle with pepper. **(Low fat and very low carb)**

Roasted Red Pepper Tapas

Tapas are traditional Spanish bar snacks. Here's a quick, easy adaptation.

2 teaspoons olive oil
1 medium onion, coarsely chopped
One 7- to 8-ounce jar roasted red bell peppers, drained and chopped
$^1\!/_2$ cup chopped and pitted kalamata olives
1 tablespoon balsamic vinegar
Sixteen $^1\!/_2$-inch slices French bread

▶ Heat the oil in a small skillet over medium-high heat. Add the onion and stir for 3 minutes. Add the peppers, olives, and vinegar, and mix well. Cook and stir for 3–4 minutes, or until the oil is evaporated. Remove from the heat. Place the bread slices on a cookie sheet. Broil 4 to 6 inches from the heat source for about 5 minutes, or until lightly toasted on both sides. To serve, spread the pepper mixture on the toast. **(Very low fat and very low carb)**

THE "DOER"
OATH FOR HEALTH

I respect my body and always provide it with the necessary exercise and nutrition it needs to make me a stronger and healthier person. I enjoy living a healthy life and truly believe I am a better person because of my dedication to myself. I *think* great thoughts, I *say* great words, and I *do* great things. I truly enjoy each day because it provides me with physical and mental challenges that condition me to become a stronger human being. I realize that the healthier, stronger, and more energetic I become, the more productive and successful I become. I realize that by making myself a better person, I am also making others around me better at the same time. My contributions to myself positively influence my world and the world around me!

I'M A DOER.™

"Doer" Testimonials

From: Dr. James Stoxen, Chiropractor
Date: Sunday, 30 December 2001

Dear John:

I have you to thank for inspiring me to take charge of my life. Becoming a DOER helped me get my life back in balance!

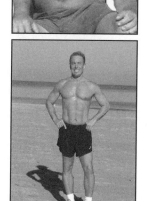

To own and operate a business requires huge amounts of physical and emotional energy! But so many professionals sacrifice health as they're striving for their wealth. At forty I was over 50 pounds overweight, not a good condition to be in either personally or professionally!

I am a health care professional who runs a therapeutic clinic and speaks to "live" audiences on a weekly basis. Having a healthy image is essential for leadership and to build a solid successful business. It wasn't helping my image or my business being so terribly out of shape. I knew I needed to make a change, and I knew I needed to start respecting my health.

Listening to you inspired me to become a DOER! After losing 50 pounds in just a few short months, *I look better than I ever did and am healthier and more energetic than ever, with a positive image fueled with loads of confidence!* Life is easier now both personally and professionally. I carry and present myself both in public and with my patients with incredible energy! I now have properly aligned my health goals to be back in balance with my financial, family, and spiritual goals.

Leaders need balance in their lives! When you are overweight and out of shape, you cannot have balance. There are no more excuses to being mentally and physically out of shape. John Abdo's guidance has literally saved my life and changed it in such remarkable ways. I now look forward to tomorrow!

A New DOER!
James Stoxen, D.C.
Evergreen Park, Illinois

From: Sherrie Crider
Date: Sunday, 16 December 2001

Dear John:

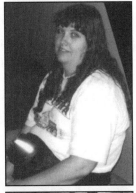

I am twenty-nine years old, 5 feet 6 inches tall, and I topped out at 214 pounds. My chest was 46½ inches, my waist was 45 inches, and my lower stomach and hips measured a total of 47 inches around! I started your routine on November 2, and ever since I have had more energy and felt as great as I did when I was a teenager! My whole attitude is better, and I thank you for it.

I want you to know that you've been a real lifesaver for me. I mean that in the literal sense. I have obstructive sleep apnea, and I was actually suffocating myself while I sleep. I blacked out while driving one day, and that is how I ended up at my doctor's office. To make a long story short, you have helped keep me alive, and I have four other people who also want to thank you. That is my husband, my ten-year-old daughter, my eight-year-old son, and my six-year-old son. Thank you from all of us.

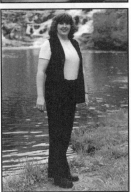

Staying committed to being a DOER, I have now lost over 50 pounds of body fat and, brace yourself for this one . . . have lost 10½ inches off my waistline!!!! I feel awesome!! I went out to purchase my first new outfit today for my husband's Christmas party that is tomorrow night. I want to look my best for him. The ladies at the clothing store asked me what size pants I thought I would need. I said that I was a 16/18 when I started my diet and exercise so I have no idea what I'd fit into now. They started out by handing me size 14's, then they went down to a 12, and then I was handed a 10!!!!!!!!!! No squeezing, no sucking in my belly . . . nothing. The pants went on smoothly and zipped right up!

I have been so excited! I feel GREAT!!!! Not only do I feel wonderful for myself but the enjoyment I am now able to provide to my family is so satisfying because I am more "fun" to be with, and I'm not sleeping and tired all the time!

Thanks, John. You are awesome!

SHERRIE
Winona, Missouri

Appendix:
Resource Guide

Online Resources

John Abdo (www.johnabdo.com): All Abdo, all the time.

American Holistic Health Organization (www.ahha.org): A Web site from the leading wellness organization. You will find many useful self-help articles, holistic practitioners, and resource lists.

Doc of Texas (www.mdmuscle.org): This site is dedicated to revealing technology, medicine, and science pertaining to hormone/medicinal intervention, behavior modification, and physician guidance.

Fitness Link (www.fitnesslink.com): Informational Web site with free and paid membership areas. Pages carry a wealth of carefully researched articles on body, mind, diet, career, men's and women's fitness issues, etc. Also contains quizzes, interesting facts, and self-assessments.

HealthWorld Online (www.healthy.net): A vast Web site covering many aspects of wellness, fitness, nutrition, and health. There are many links to such topics as nutrition, healthy travel, healthy shopping, and children's issues. Related products are sold via the site, and a free newsletter is available.

International Sports Sciences Association (www.issaonline.com): Geared toward personal trainers, health and fitness professionals and those seeking certification and continuing education programs in the health and fitness fields. Includes a "trainer locator" for individuals interested in enlisting the assistance of a personal trainer.

Jay Robb Enterprises (*www.jayrobb.com*): This site offers a unique and versatile approach to getting fit, lean, and muscular with free recipes, newsletters, and more!

Life Extension Foundation (www.lef.org): The world's largest organization dedicated to finding scientific methods of preventing and treating disease, aging, and death. In addition to developing unique disease treatment protocols, the foundation funds pioneering scientific research aimed at achieving an indefinitely extended healthy human life span. This site contains a nutritional product section, breaking news, cutting-edge research, and live chats with experts.

LosingWeight.com (losingweight.com): This self-described Weightloss Superstore offers everything from educational materials to fitness equipment. Lots of products to choose from.

Muscle and Fitness Magazine (www.muscleandfitness.com): Joe Weider's award-winning publication is now available online. Learn the secrets to building a stronger and more muscular body with diet, sports medicine, exercise physiology, and much more.

Planet Muscle (www.planetmuscle.com): This online magazine has many articles related to bodybuilding, ranging from programs for gaining muscle to information on hormones to a multitude of workout routines.

Pro-Trainer Online (www.protraineronline.com): "The Strongest Fitness Magazine on the Net." This Web site is dedicated to all aspects of strength training. The articles cover traditional topics such as nutrition as well as more diverse topics such as yoga. Also contains The Very Good Question Section with a lot of . . . well . . . very good questions (and answers).

SpeakersForHealth.Com (www.speakersforhealth.com): A great source for professional speakers on health care and wellness.

Thane International (www.thane.com): This leading direct marketing firm offers a multitude of health, fitness, beauty, and weight loss products, including the AB-DOer.

Phone Numbers, Postal and E-Mail Addresses

International Sports Sciences Association
Fitness training certification and educational courses
(800) 892-4772
3920 B State Street
Santa Barbara, CA 93105

Life Extension Foundation
Anti-aging foundation
(800) 841-5433
2490 Griffin Road
Fort Lauderdale, Fl 33312

Dr. Michael C. Scally
Hormone and medicinal intervention, behavior modification, and
physician guidance
(888) 673-0077
E-mail: docoftexas@docoftexas.net
8707 Katy Freeway, Suite C
Houston, Texas 77024

Dr. Bernard Stevens
Hormonal evaluations, body compositions
bbstev@hotmail.com

Suggested Readings

Abdo, John, and Ken Dachman. *Body Engineering* (New York: Perigee Publishing, 1997).

Gastelu, Daniel, and Fred Hatfield. *Dynamic Nutrition for Maximum Performance* (New York: Putnam Publishing Group, 1997).

Goldman, Robert, with Ronald Klatz and Lisa Berger. *Brain-Fitness: Anti-Aging Strategies for Achieving Super Mind Power* (New York: Doubleday, 1999).

Robb, Jay. *The Fat-Burning Diet* (Santee, Calif.: Loving Health Publications, 1996).

Ulene, Art. *The NutriBase Complete Book of Food Counts* (Wayne, N.J.: Avery Penguin Putnam, 1996).

Weider, Betty, and Joe Weider. *The Weider Body Book* (Chicago: Contemporary Books, 1984).

Weider, Joe, with Bill Renolds. *The Best of Joe Weider's Flex Nutrition and Training Programs* (Chicago: Contemporary Books, 1990).

Wilmore, Jack H. *Physiology of Sport and Exercise* (Champaign, Ill.: Human Kinetics Publishers, 1999).

Wilmore, Jack H., and David Costill. *Training for Sport and Activity* (Dubuque, Iowa: William C. Brown Company, 1988).

John Abdo's Products and Services

Exercise Equipment

The AB-DOer is the world's first midsection aerobic machine that was invented by John Abdo. Millions of people worldwide are successfully using *The AB-DOer* to lose fat around their midsections while strengthening the muscles of their spinal columns. Voted the No. 1 product of the year in 2001, *The AB-DOer* has revolutionized the health and fitness industry.

Total Body Doer is a complete health club of exercise equipment built into one machine. Co-developed by John Abdo, this machine offers dozens of exercises for the upper body, lower body, and midsection.

The Orbitrek is the ultimate in-home elliptical steppers. This remarkable zero-impact aerobic machine combines upper-body pumping with a revolutionary lower-body elliptical action. You can burn 4 to 5 times as many calories using the *Orbitrek* as on a treadmill, bike, or stair climber. Lifetime warranty.

Video and Audio Tapes

Walk-A-Dobics is a set of instructional video tapes created by John Abdo that offers a fun yet challenging "indoor" walking program! The three videos include a *Metabolic Stimulator* program, *The Fat Attack* video, and a healthy breathing and stretching video called *Oxywalk*. As a bonus, *Walk-A-Dobics* also includes a

20-minute motivational audiotape and a Nutrition Guide that addresses fat weight loss and healthy eating suggestions.

John Abdo's Vital Living from the Inside Out is a 4-cassette audio program that clarifies the myths and uncovers the realities of living a better, more productive, more successful life. Written and hosted by John Abdo, this series covers success-proven strategies for improving physical and mental fitness.

John Abdo's "No-Excuses Workout" is an instructional workout video that can be performed anywhere and at any time, hence *no excuses*. This routine is based on a combination of strength training, muscle toning, fat burning, cardiovascular, and flexibility movements all in one routine that takes only seven minutes.

Nutritionals

John Abdo formulates and endorses a variety of nutritional supplements that improve health, enhance performance, boost metabolism, reduce body fat, improve appearance, stimulate sexual functions, and develop overall well-being. Realizing that nutrition is an ever-growing science, John Abdo has a mission of staying with or ahead of nutritional technological advancements, and so information regarding current food and nutritional recommendations can be found on John's Web site at johnabdo.com.

Acknowledgments

To my beloved father, Donald John Abdo, who made (not purchased) my first set of dumbbells and introduced me to the world of physical fitness.

To my beloved mother, Alice Jane Abdo, who has made my life extremely fulfilling with her endless love and support.

To my beloved girlfriend and best friend, Linda Marie Lee, for her immense understanding and encouragement.

To my younger brother, Steven Salem Abdo, who has endured a great deal of pain submitting to my exercise and routine experimentations during my formative years as a fitness authority. Sorry, Steve.

To Dr. Kenneth Dachman for assisting me in making these pages possible and for his immense contributions to the psychological aspects of fitness, obesity, and health.